Evolution of Epidemiologic Ideas

Annotated Readings on Concepts and Methods

Sander Greenland, Editor

Evolution of Epidemiologic Ideas: Annotated Readings on Concepts and Methods

Edited by

Sander Greenland
Division of Epidemiology
University of California School of Public Health
Los Angeles, California

Epidemiology Resources Inc.

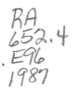

Table of Contents

Preface

In the Fall of 1984, Nancy Dreyer of Epidemiology Resources Inc. invited me to prepare an historical anthology of writings in epidemiologic methods. The resulting collection covers two broad areas: Issues in Causal Inference, and Developments in Theory and Quantitative Methods. I have given each part its own preface, and supplied each article with a brief introduction. Here I preface elements common to both parts.

For manifold reasons, I chose to restrict the selections to roughly the three decades following World War II. Earlier works were difficult to obtain, often contained lengthy digressions, and many were written in an archaic style with which I had little patience. Most importantly, I had no resources for a scholarly search of prewar literature. At the other end, works written within the last ten years have hardly been around long enough to be termed historical, and my projection of their ultimate status is heavily biased by my personal impressions of many of the authors (the same can be said, I admit, of my selections from the 1970's).

The period actually covered, 1946–1977, encompasses most of what I perceive as two "golden eras" of epidemiologic development. The first, roughly 1946–1966, saw the creation of a foundation for modern epidemiologic methods, including the development of basic methods for relative risk estimation, in parallel with the first major epidemiologic studies of chronic diseases. The second, roughly 1967–1981, saw the construction of a theoretical framework for epidemiologic methods, including clarification of concepts such as confounding and interaction, in parallel with the emergence of the case-control design as the primary epidemiologic method in cancer research. The present collection is too limited to convey this picture clearly, but I hope it gives the reader a fair idea of the origins of some now-established methods, and some flavor for the often ragged pattern of development and dissemination of ideas.

The period covered by this volume is too recent to assure complete consensus over the historical importance of most of my selections. There are, however, many articles that may be of debatable importance but that I would want to see read as part of the historical record, if only for fun (the Popper debate is an example of this type of reading). My apologies to those colleagues whose favorites were omitted.

Editor's Acknowledgments

I would like to thank Charles Poole and James Schlesselman for their suggestions for readings, and their comments on my text (though there remain important points of disagreement among all three of us); Nancy Dreyer and Kenneth Rothman, for suggesting and encouraging this project; the faculty, staff, and students of the Epidemiology and Biometry Section, School of Public Health and Tropical Medicine, University of Sydney, for providing a most pleasant and stimulating environment for producing this book during my Fall 1985 sabbatical; Virginia Hansen and Evalon Witt of UCLA, for helping prepare the original text; and Margaret Satterfield and Philip Setel of ERI, for their work in obtaining reprint permission and preparing the book for press.

Publisher's Acknowledgments

We are grateful for permission to reprint the following papers:

Hill, Austin Bradford. Observation and experiment. New England Journal of Medicine, 1953. Reproduced by the permission of the New England Journal of Medicine. Cornfield, Jerome. Statistical relationships and proof in medicine. American Statistician, 1954. Reproduced by permission of The American Statistical Association. Hill, Austin Bradford. The environment and disease: association or causation? Proceedings of the Royal Society of Medicine, 1965. Reproduced by permission of the Royal Society of Medicine. Sartwell, Philip E. "On the methodology of investigations of etiologic factors in chronic diseases"–further comments. Journal of Chronic Diseases, 1960. Reproduced by permission of the author and Pergamon Press, Ltd. MacMahon, Brian and Thomas F Pugh. Causes and entities of disease. In *Preventive Medicine,* DW Clark and B MacMahon eds., 1967. Reproduced by permission of Brian MacMahon and Little, Brown and Co. Miettinen, Olli. Confounding and effect-modification. American Journal of Epidemiology, 1974. Reproduced by permission of the author and the American Journal of Epidemiology. Rothman, Kenneth J. Causes. American Journal of Epidemiology, 1976. Reproduced by permission of the author and the American Journal of Epidemiology. Buck, Carol Popper's philosophy for epidemiologists. International Journal of Epidemiology, 1975. Reproduced from the International Journal of Epidemiology by permission of the author and the Oxford University Press. Replies by: AM Davies, A Smith, A Creese, R Peto, C Buck. Reproduced from the International Journal of Epidemiology by permission of the Oxford University Press. Jacobsen, M. Against Popperized epidemiology. International Journal of Epidemiology, 1976. Reproduced from the International Journal of Epidemiology by permission of the author and the Oxford University Press. Susser, Mervyn. Judgment and causal inference: criteria in epidemiologic studies. American Journal of Epidemiology, 1977. Reproduced by permission of the author and the American Journal of Epidemiology. Berkson, Joseph. Limitations of the application of fourfold table analysis to hospital data. Biometrics, 1946; 2:339–343. Reproduced with permission from The Biometric Society. Simpson, EH. The interpretation of interaction in contingency tables. Journal of the Royal Statistical Society, 1951. Reproduced by permission of the Royal Statistical Society. Woolf, Barnet. On estimating the relation between blood group and disease. Annals of Human Genetics, 1955. Reproduced from the Annals of Human Genetics by permission of the Cambridge University Press. Mantel, Nathan and William Haenszel. Statistical aspects of the analysis of data from retrospective studies of disease. Journal of the National Cancer Institute, 1959. Reproduced by permission of Nathan Mantel. Miettinen, Olli S. Components of the crude risk ratio. American Journal of Epidemiology, 1972. Reproduced by permission of the author and the American Journal of Epidemiology. Cornfield, Jerome. Joint dependence of risk of coronary heart disease on serum cholesterol and systolic blood pressure. Federation Proceedings, 1962. Reproduced by permission of The Federation of American Societies for Experimental Biology. Gordon, Tavia. Hazards in the use of the logistic function. Journal of Chronic Diseases, 1974. Reproduced by permission of Pergamon Press, Ltd. Sheehe, Paul R. Dynamic risk analysis in retrospective matched pair studies of disease. Biometrics, 1962; 18:323–341. Reproduced with permission from the author and The Biometric Society. Miettinen, Olli. Estimability and estimation in case-referent studies. American Journal of Epidemiology, 1976. Reproduced by permission of the author and the American Journal of Epidemiology.

Part I

Issues in Causal Inference

Part I is meant to serve as a source of articles that reflected or influenced epidemiologists' views on causal inference during the post-1945 era. The first four articles (from 1953–65) arose from early debates over fundamentals of causal inference in epidemiology and public health. This literature tended to regard a causal inference as the evolutionary outcome of a series of careful judgments of evidence, and these judgments were based on criteria that for the most part were neither necessary nor sufficient. The last four articles (from 1967–1976) reflect a more formal and quantitatively oriented view of causal inference in epidemiology that emerged from Harvard in the 1960's. This literature tended to regard a causal inference as a (possibly temporary) construct necessitated by failure to find a plausible alternative explanation (e.g., confounding) of an association. The latter orientation is closer to the Popperian view of science, a debate on which is reprinted here. Part I closes with some learned reflections on the matter by a renowned contributor to epidemiology.

I-1.

Austin Bradford Hill: Observation and Experiment.
New England Journal of Medicine 1953; 248:995–1001.

My first choice for this section, Bradford Hill's "Observation and Experiment," is at once a product of its time and filled with advice as relevant today as in 1953. At that time there was still much skepticism concerning the value of nonexperimental (or "observational") research in epidemiology. Hill's comments on the subject came in the midst of an important controversy over the role of cigarette smoking in the etiology of human lung cancer. Bear in mind that when Hill wrote, no cohort studies of the matter had been completed, and the causal nature of the cigarette-cancer association was still contested by many respectable scientists, including no less a figure than Sir Ronald Fisher.

Hill defended nonexperimental methods in a constructive and instructive manner, presenting the problems we would today label as confounding, information bias, and selection bias as part of the researcher's task to solve, rather than as insurmountable flaws inherent in all nonexperimental research. One of the foremost medical statisticians of his day, he also took care to point out the danger of substituting statistics for thought in the analysis and presentation of data, as his discussion of field experiments so well illustrates. This message is, I believe, as timely today as ever. Finally, Hill recognized the importance of the interplay of imaginative theorization and logical deduction in research—a theme that we will encounter again in the readings on Popper's philosophy for epidemiologists.

The New England
Journal of Medicine

Copyright, 1953, by the Massachusetts Medical Society

Volume 248   JUNE 11, 1953   Number 24

OBSERVATION AND EXPERIMENT*

A. Bradford Hill, C.B.E., D.Sc., Ph.D.†

LONDON, ENGLAND

TWO years ago, in his Cutter Lecture, one of my predecessors pointed out that the object of any science is "the accumulation of systematized verifiable knowledge," and that this is to be achieved through "observation, experiment and thought" — the last including both criticism and imagination. He then added, "the use of the experimental method has brilliant discoveries to its credit, whereas the method of observation has achieved little."[1] This dictum must surely prove, at least at first sight, more than a little disconcerting to the exponent of preventive medicine. In dealing with the characteristics of human populations, in sorting out the features of the environment that are detrimental from those that are beneficial, he does not often find it easy to experiment. The method of observation frequently plays a large part in the particular study of mankind that is his prerogative. Is it, then, quite so useless? Must he give it up as merely a time-wasting hobby?

Looking farther back in time I found that these questions had been considered, as indeed I had expected, by my statistical forebears and teachers in Great Britain. They did not perhaps have quite so pessimistic an outlook as the one I have quoted above, but they certainly did not underrate the difficulties of the observational approach or overlook the value of the experimental method. Thus, in 1924, Yule's[2] view was that the student of social facts could not experiment but had to deal with circumstances operating entirely beyond his control; he must accept records simply of what has happened. He wrote:

> The expert in public health, for example, must take the records of deaths as they occur, and endeavour as best he can to interpret, say, the varying incidence of death on different districts. Clearly this is a very difficult matter...The purpose of *experiment* is to replace these highly complex tangles of causation, [and] the more perfect the experiment — the more nearly the experimental ideal is attained — the less is the influence of disturbing causes, and the less necessary the use of statistical methods.

*The Cutter Lecture on Preventive Medicine, delivered at the Harvard School of Public Health, March 25, 1953.

†Professor of medical statistics and director of the Department of Medical Statistics and Epidemiology, London School of Hygiene and Tropical Medicine; honorary director, Statistical Research Unit of the Medical Research Council, England.

Greenwood[3] has a characteristic passage, which I quote in full since I believe that the part of it that has no close bearing on my present thesis will nevertheless more than bear repetition today;

> My conception of the statistical method in medicine has changed in the last 20 years; this is especially so with regard to the bearing of statistical method upon experiment. I used to see in the statistician the critic of the laboratory worker: it is a rôle which is gratifying to youthful vanity, for it is so easy to cheat oneself into the belief that the critic has some intellectual superiority over the criticised. I do not think even now that statistical criticism of laboratory investigations is useless, but I attach enormously more value to direct collaboration, the making of statistical experiments, and the permeation of statistical research with the experimental spirit.

The last words — written nearly thirty years ago — are, I suggest, the operative clause in the present setting — the permeation of statistical research with the experimental spirit. Although, as Yule said, facts must often, inevitably, be accepted as they occur, one does not have merely to accept facts as they are reported. One need not accept as final what some third party can give, or chooses to give — for example, a registrar-general or a census bureau. Such reported observations may, of course, prove to be a most valuable indicator of a problem; they may be, thereby, the starting point of research. But when the pattern of cause and effect is complicated they are often not likely to provide a solution. The methods of partial correlation, enthusiastically accepted a quarter of a century ago, no longer seem to have an "unlimited power to penetrate the secrets of nature."[4] One must go seek more facts, paying less attention to technics of handling the data and far more to the development and perfection of methods of obtaining them. In so doing one must have the experimental approach firmly in mind. In other words, can observations be made in such a way as to fulfil, as far as possible, experimental requirements?

Ancient Observation (the Cholera)

It was in this way, nearly a hundred years ago, that John Snow approached his problem, not only as an incomparable master of logical deduction from observations but also, it should be noted, as the constructor of observations. To recapitulate briefly, his opening arguments are based on vital statistics of the different areas of London. Using the deaths given in the first report of the Metropolitan Sanitary Commission (1847), he first shows the excessive mortality from cholera that in the epidemic of 1832 befell the districts supplied by the Southwark Water Works, a company that drew its water from the Thames at London Bridge and provided worse water, according to Snow, than any other in the metropolis. Even the order of precedence between a flea and a louse is sometimes, it appears, of importance. A death rate from cholera of 11 per 1000 inhabitants stands out starkly amidst the rates of 2, 3 and 4 for other districts of the city, but clearly that unenviable record might be explicable in terms of some quite different local characteristic. The evidence gives a lead but no more. The case is somewhat, but not at all convincingly, strengthened by the events of 1849. The highest mortality rates from cholera were again consistently to be found in the districts supplied by the Southwark Company (now combined with the South London Water Company to form the Southwark and Vauxhall) and also in those served by the Lambeth Company; both companies drew their water from the Thames in its most contaminated reaches. In 1853 there begins to appear reason to sit up and even to take notice. The Lambeth Company had removed its works from central London to Thames Ditton, where the river was wholly free from the sewage of the metropolis; the Southwark and Vauxhall Company continued to prescribe for its customers the mixture as before. In the 12 subdistricts served by the latter 192 persons died of cholera in the epidemic of 1853 — with 168,000 persons living the crude rate is thus 114 per 100,000. In 16 subdistricts served by both companies 182 perons died; among 301,000 living, that is a rate of 60 per 100,000. In three subdistricts of 15,000 persons served only by the Lambeth Company no deaths from cholera were reported.

So far do the statistical observations run; so far but not far enough. On that showing alone one might even hesitate to accept Snow's "very strong evidence" against the water supply. He himself was indeed of that mind, for "the question," he observed, "does not end here" (he had no intention of letting it end .there). It was not said without reason that wherever cholera was visitant there was he in the midst. He noted that the Southwark and Vauxhall and Lambeth companies were competitors so that in some subdistricts the pipes of each went down all the streets and into nearly all the courts and alleys:

Each Company supplies both rich and poor, both large houses and small...No fewer than 300,000 people of both sexes, of every age and occupation, and of every rank and station, from gentlefolk down to the very poor, were divided into two groups without their choice, and, in most cases, without their knowledge; one group being supplied with water containing the sewage of London, and, amongst it, what-

ever might have come from the cholera patients, the other group having water quite free from such impurity.

Here, then, was an unwitting experiment on the grandest scale, and Snow set himself to learn its results.

In 1854, with one medical man to assist him, up and down the streets, courts and alleys of South London he tramped in the summer's sun, learning for every cholera death the water supply of the household. Thus, by personal, persistent and accurate field work were the basic vital statistics infinitely strengthened. In 40,000 houses served by the Southwark and Vauxhall Company 286 fatal attacks were found in the first four weeks of the epidemic of 1854 — 71 deaths per 10,000 households; in 26,000 houses served by the Lambeth Company 14 fatal attacks were found — only 5 deaths per 10,000 households. In such a way was observation successfully added to observation to form a coherent and convincing whole.

It might be argued that Snow was lucky in having at hand a natural "experiment." Perhaps he was. But such "experiments" or, at the least, effective "controls" would not, I believe, really prove to be so rare if one invariably cast one's eyes round for them after vital statistics, or similar observations, had given an appropriate lead.

Certainly, in the famous Broad Street Pump outbreak of cholera no experiment offered. Its story is too well known to need any detailed reference here, but having brought Snow into my picture, I could not bear to pass it by wholly unsung. It is not so much for persuading the local board of guardians to remove the handle of the pump that Snow here deserves credit — though for this alone it is often paid to him. In fact either through the flight of the terrified population from the stricken area (and Snow himself says that "in less than 6 days the most afflicted streets were deserted by more than three-quarters of their inhabitants") or through natural epidemiologic causes, the outbreak had been steeply declining for five or six days before the well was thus put out of action. That "experiment" provides no useful evidence.

It is again in the field work that his strength lies: the map showing the concentration of deaths around the pump with their number diminishing greatly, or ceasing altogether, at each point where it became decidedly nearer to send to another pump; the demonstration of the escape of the inmates of the workhouse, which had its own well, and, similarly, of the 70 workmen in the brewery who knew better than to drink water — or if somehow driven to do so drew from a well within the brewery. And the striking individual histories, the most conclusive of which Sherlock Holmes might well have called "the curious case of the Hampstead widow." In the weekly return of births and deaths of September 9 published by the Registrar-General of England and

Wales there appeared the following entry: "At West End [Hampstead], on 2nd September, the widow of a percussion-cap maker, aged 59 years, diarrhoea two hours, cholera epidemica sixteen hours." (The times refer to the duration of the fatal illness, then — and again now — entered by the medical practitioner upon the certificate of cause of death.) One of the factories in Broad Street made percussion caps, but on inquiry Snow found that the widow had not been in the neighborhood for many months. However, she still preferred the water from the pump to that of the more salubrious neighborhood to which she had retired, and she commissioned a carter who drove daily between the two points to bring her a large bottle. The bottle was duly delivered on August 31. She drank of it and died two days later. A niece on a visit to her likewise drank of it. She then returned to her home in Islington, where she died of cholera. There was no cholera extant in either neighborhood.

To digress for a moment, there was at least one other person who drank of that bottle. The story here is, perhaps, less well known. The first medical officer of health for Hampstead (now one of the metropolitan boroughs of London) dictated as an old man in 1889 some recollections under the title of "The Sanitary Experiences of Charles F. J. Lord, M.R.C.S." It is now held in manuscript in the Hampstead Public Library but was privately printed for circulation among the old man's friends. There is a copy in the library of the Surgeon General in Washington under the title, "Jottings: Some experience with reflections derived through life and work in Hampstead from 1827 to 1877" (Pamphlet Vol. 3807). Lord himself died before making final corrections of the proofs. On pages 36 and 37 of the printed version the following passage is included:

A memorable case of what we may consider an imported cause of disease happened at West End; Mrs. Eley Mother of the renowned firm "Eley Brothers" had lived in Broad Street Soho, and had drunk with glorification from a deep well there situated. On leaving London, she had a big stone bottle brought daily for the use of herself at West End. Summoned hastily to see the old lady I found her in the early stage of Cholera — remedies were unavailing, though solicitously applied in every way by a daughter and one of her sons. A consultation with the highly esteemed Dr. Farre ensued, the Patient never rallied, died that night. The cause of the disease at that time was never suspected; it was proved afterwards by the untiring investigations of Dr. Snow, that the water from the Broad Street well was contaminated and produced the disease; a sort of practical joke arose among the Teetotalers of the Broad Street district; those who stuck to the Porter especially those of the Brewery were rarely victims to the disease while those who drank the water fell fast around. I myself while attending closely on the old lady, as also was her daughter, was much troubled with Diarrhoea having unsuspiciously sipped some of the imported water. This insipient [sic] stage of Cholera soon passed away, in the absence of full or renewed doses.

Here, then, to return to my thesis, is a masterpiece — many persons would say the masterpiece — of observation and logical inference, made many years before the discovery of the vibrio of cholera.

It shows — as many other examples have shown — that the highest returns can be reaped by imagination in combination with a logical and critical mind, a spice of ingenuity coupled with an eye for the simple and humdrum, and a width of vision in the pursuit of facts that is allied with an attention to detail that is almost nauseating.

MODERN OBSERVATION (RUBELLA)

A modern example of acute observation lies in the story of rubella in pregnancy unfolded, almost a hundred years later, in Australia. Again, the story is too well known to need retelling, but it has a facet perhaps less familiar and yet of great interest to the student of public health — in other words, to the observer of group phenomena. It might well be that the congenital defects observed in Australia in the years 1938 to 1941 were something new in medicine, that the rubella epidemic was of a particular virulence, or that the virus had acquired some unusual characteristic at that time. Indeed, there is so much folklore attached to events in pregnancy that if the effects of German measles were an old phenomenon one might possibly have expected to find some old-wives' tale concerning it. I know of none in Britain. That the story was not, however, new in Australia is strongly indicated by the statistical observations marshaled by Lancaster.[5] In each of the reports on the Australian censuses of 1911, 1921 and 1933 there is a section that deals with the enumerated prevalence of blindness and deaf-mutism. The incidence of the latter is revealing; it shows a maximum in each census corresponding to persons born in the years 1896-1900.

At the census of 1911 the peak lay in the age group from ten to fourteen, and the statistician, writes Lancaster, "was inclined to ascribe the maximum to the more complete enumeration of the deaf at the school ages"; most observers would, I suspect, have taken that view. When, however, in 1921, the peak shifted to the age group twenty to twenty-four the statistician considered epidemic disease as a possible cause. He suggested that the increased incidence of deafness at certain ages might synchronize with the occurrence of such illnesses as "scarlet fever, diphtheria, measles, and whooping cough." In the report on the census of 1933 infective disease was again discussed. But the lead given by the somewhat crude vital statistics was not, it appears, followed up at the time. Lancaster himself has followed it up — in 1951 and therefore, of course, after the clinical observations of 1938-41 — by examining the dates of birth of children admitted to institutions for the deaf and dumb. He finds, to take a single example, that of those admitted in New South Wales 15 were born in 1898 and 16 in 1900. For the intermediate year 1899 the figure soared to 70. Furthermore, these 70 are not evenly spread throughout the year but are concentrated in the months

998   THE NEW ENGLAND JOURNAL OF MEDICINE   June 11, 1953

of April to September. On such evidence, marshaled in detail and with skill, Lancaster concludes that "deafness has appeared in epidemic form in Australia in the past, notably among children born in 1899, 1916, 1924, 1925 and in 1938-41" and that "there is some presumptive evidence that all these epidemics, with the exception of that in 1916, were caused by antecedent epidemics of rubella." It seems so easy *now*, he rightly observes, to suggest a causal relation; it is always easy to be wise after the event. Nevertheless, there was at least a legible scrawl on the wall — additional and accurate data were there for the seeking and, once sought, offered a clear case for a carefully designed field inquiry. The combined observational and statistical approach could have won the day; it could have won it quite a long time ago.

CANCER OF THE LUNG

This approach seems to me to be the only one possible in another matter of community concern today — the etiology of carcinoma of the lung. The starting point is as usual the national registration system. "It is sometimes asked," says Stocks,[6] "how statistics can cure disease," and he suggests that one may counter the question by another question: "how many researches which have led to real advances in Medicine would ever have been started had there not first been some statistics to suggest that here was a problem to be investigated?" In this particular instance it is, of course, admitted that skill in, and modern adjuncts to, diagnosis make more than dubious the whole gamut of changes that the system of vital statistics reveals. But there is, in my opinion, more than enough evidence to regard some of that change as real and to justify a search for a cause of a truly rising mortality in England and Wales. Aided and abetted by the Medical Research Council, Doll and I set about that search in 1947. Our aim was to make the field observations mirror an experimental design as nearly as possible. For each patient with cancer of the lung we sought a "control" patient with some other disease — a patient of the same sex, of the same age group, in the same hospital at or about the same time, but otherwise chosen at random. In other words, we sought, as in an experiment, to limit the variables. We limited them, too, not only in this way but also by employing, in history taking, only a few skilled interviewers, each armed with a prescribed set of questions. We made, of course, no frontal attack upon smoking, which in our original questionnaire formed but one section out of nine — eleven questions out of nearly fifty.

Having admitted to a questionnaire of that magnitude I shall take this opportunity to defend myself. For I have been reported as having advocated, before a conference on the application of scientific methods to industrial and service medicine, "that nobody should be subjected to more than five ques-

tions."[7] I am, indeed, in favor of shorter and brighter forms but not always to that extent. What I said on that occasion about the problems of making observations of any value, was this: "broadly speaking, of any twenty questions asked in a field survey not more than five should be put to the surveyed, and not less than fifteen should be put to the surveyor by himself before he enters the field or, indeed, ventures to look over the gate."[8] In other words, I maintained, though doubtless somewhat clumsily, that one may ask as many questions as one believes useful — so long as the ratio one to the surveyed and three to the surveyor is maintained throughout. A basic query in the latter group will be, in every case, "is this question really necessary?" It is surprising how often that will effectively keep down the number incorporated.

On the other hand the observational approach has perhaps been somewhat discredited by a too frequent failure to keep down that number, a pathetically notable lack of the critical and imaginative thought that, as Sinclair noted, must be an integral part of the scientific method, — in other words, and more briefly, too few ideas chasing too many forms. That evil is, of course, no prerogative of the United States of America, but I cannot refrain from citing from Eric Linklater's[9] delectable book (that is, to an Englishman) *Juan in America*. Even twenty-two years ago he was moved to write that "the issuing of questionnaires had become a national habit, and work was provided for many people, who might otherwise never have found employment, in dealing with such returns: that is in docketing them, tabulating, copying, indexing, cross-indexing, rearranging them, according to ethnic, religious, social, geographic and other factors, and eventually composing a monograph on them for the Library of Congress." Perhaps Americans were quicker off the mark. I would, however, warn them that we on the other side of the Atlantic are not being backward and may even overtake them in these national vices and devices.

Returning to my theme it is, of course, possible that the relative absence of nonsmokers and the relative frequency of heavy smokers that Doll and I found in our patients with cancer of the lung (and that other workers have also noted) is really a function of some other difference between the two groups. We do not ourselves, for several reasons, believe that to be so, and it is certainly worth noting that patients with pulmonary cancer and controls are remarkably alike in other characteristics that we have recorded. Nevertheless, here lies, I admit, the weakness of the observational as compared with the experimental approach. With the former we can determine the most probable explanation of a contrast in our data; given the provision that we have taken sufficient care to remove disturbing causes, that probability can be very high. But with a well designed experiment it should be possible to eliminate (or allow for) nearly all disturbing causes and thus to render the interpretation of the contrast even more certain.

Yet in this particular problem what experiment can one make? We may subject mice, or other laboratory animals, to such an atmosphere of tobacco smoke that they can — like the old man in the fairy story — neither sleep nor slumber; they can neither breed nor eat. And lung cancers may or may not develop to a significant degree. What then? We may have thus strengthened the evidence, we may even have narrowed the search, but we must, I believe, invariably return to man for the final proof or proofs.

In this instance one other method of inquiry is now being applied both in the United States and the United Kingdom: a "looking-forward" investigation. Up till now investigators have taken already marked subjects — together with a control series — and have inquired into their antecedents. That has been the method not only, of course, in this particular inquiry but in many others. It is a natural approach and one likely to yield quick returns. Adult patients with peptic ulcers are questioned concerning whether they came from broken homes; those with rheumatoid arthritis are questioned on their previous shocks and ills; and the views of the victims of neurosis upon the habits of their fathers are sought. The resulting picture, the contrast between marked and unmarked, may be clear cut, and yet it may be difficult to distinguish between effects and causes, between horse and cart. Memories may well be more profound and more retentive in the "marked," and they may indeed be more highly colored — what the adult neurotic thinks of his father may not always be the truth. Even with the method at its best one can rarely hope to make a prognosis by these means, to measure the probabilities of events. But that is what is usually needed: first to observe the broken, and unbroken, home and then to record the subsequent history of its youthful inmates. That is clearly difficult to do and calls for a considerable degree of patience, which most investigators do not possess. But if the forward approach can be employed, it is, I believe, almost always the right way to go to work; in any observational inquiry its possibility should invariably be considered.

In the particular investigation that Doll and I now have under way — broadly into the deaths in the next few years of men and women on the British medical register whose smoking habits are already characterized at a defined point of time (late 1951) — it again, of course, would not follow that any association we might find between death from carcinoma of the lung (or other causes of death) and smoking habits must be a direct association. The heavy smokers may be differentiated from the light smokers in some other way, which might have some bearing on the risks of a bronchial carcinoma. We are still faced with the most probable explanation. But we may, I submit, have further narrowed the field of possible variables, of errors of omission or commission.

THE FIELD EXPERIMENT

There is today an increasing resort to the field experiment, a district, a town, a school or a factory being used as the laboratory. It is a striking development of the present age and, if the requirements of an efficient experiment can be met, a most valuable one. But those requirements *must* be met; a poor experiment serves no purpose. Yet it seems that the very magic in its name may serve to mislead those who worship at the experimental shrine.

As an example, in a recently reported study of vaccination against influenza, the subjects for inoculation were chosen on a voluntary basis and "without any great propaganda 32.8% of the total employees involved in the Survey voluntarily requested the inoculations." This one third, self-selected group is compared with the remaining two thirds, who, like Gallio, "cared for none of those things." Of the 1148 inoculated persons 10.80 per cent were attacked by influenza, and of the 2349 remaining population 15.02 per cent. The difference is "statistically significant" with a "P of 0.00567." And yet does this ritual and do all these decimal places mean anything at all? Admittedly, the technical test says that the two groups had experiences that differed by more than one would expect to occur by chance; equally, it tells nothing else. As it stands I do not myself believe that it gives any support whatever for the author's conclusion that here is evidence "strongly in favor of the immunization of large groups in industry." Yet I have no doubt that it will be cited in the literature under the caption "it has been shown by experiment."

In my view this is not an experiment at all. Some observations have been made of the recorded incidence of "influenza" in two groups. The investigator knew (and so incidentally did the two groups) that they differed in one respect — inoculation; they may well have differed in a score of others — even, for all one is told, in such simple respects as age and sex. None of the other possible variables of importance were controlled, and it is well known that in trials of vaccines a self-selected group is most unlikely to be a representative sample of the total. Field experiments are not, unfortunately, as easy to design and carry out as all that. In this particular field — vaccination against influenza — I speak with conviction, for the Medical Research Council has during the last winter carried out some experiments in industry, — trials of methodology, I should say, as much as of vaccines. We too, of course, have had to rely upon volunteers for our basic material. There is (fortunately) no other way of setting up a trial.

But the volunteers were divided at random into two groups — an inoculated group given the influenza vaccine and an inoculated group given a dummy vaccine. We had their general consent to that procedure, but in the individual case it was unknown. It was also unknown to the medical practitioner diagnosing such illnesses as occurred — influenza, possibly influenza and other diseases. In such ways we have endeavored to equalize our groups *de novo* — to eliminate bias from the subsquent observations. Whether, having to cast our epidemic net wide, we have succeeded in obtaining accurate and comparable records from a score of factories and still more doctors remains to be seen. Such experiments involving human beings are, I repeat, not easy to carry out; they are, as a rule, costly. Yet in relation to the returns rendered they are relatively cheap. A well designed plan may in a few months, or years, forestall years or decades of indeterminate, unplanned observation.

CONCLUSION

There is one thread that runs — or it might be more accurate to say wanders — through this lecture. I have been unable — even if I would — to conceal my preference in preventive medicine for the experimental approach. At the same time that preference does not lead me to repudiate or even, I hope, to underrate the claims of accurate and designed observations. But I would place all the emphasis at my command upon those adjectives. In this field of preventive medicine I share, on the whole, the view regarding the curative aspects recently expressed by Platt,[10] professor of medicine in the University of Manchester. Records in clinical research are likely, he suggests, to be disappointing;

Unless they have been kept with an end in view, as part of a planned experiment...Clinical experiment need not mean the subjection of patients to uncomfortable procedures of doubtful value or benefit. It means the planning of a line of action and the recording of observations designed to withstand critical analysis and give the answer to a clinical problem. It is an attitude of mind.

In appropriately exploiting that attitude of mind one may well need, in this age of technicalities, close and constant collaboration. Today, as Joseph Garland[11] pointed out in this city of Boston, "the mathematics of research has expressed itself in a multiplicity of graphs, charts and tables with the aid of which the average reader at a quick glance can often learn next to nothing." The biostatistician must therefore acquire a taste for lying down with the epidemiologist, and the bacteriologist with the medical officer of health (I speak in fables).

There are, of course, no grounds for antagonism between experiment and observation. The former, indeed, depends on observation but of a type that has the good fortune to be controlled at the experimenter's will. In the world of public health and preventive medicine each will — or should — con-

stantly react beneficially upon the other. Observation in the field suggests experiment; the experiment leads back to more, and better defined, observations. However that may be, it is difficult to see how one can wholly, or ever, escape from Alexander Pope's epigram. How else but by observation upon man himself being born, living and dying, can one set about the solution of such problems as prematurity and stillbirth at one end of life and cancer and coronary thrombosis at the other? However tangled the skein of causation one must, at least at first, try to unravel it in vivo. As Pickering[12] has said: "Any work which seeks to elucidate the cause of disease, the mechanism of disease, the cure of disease, or the prevention of disease, must begin and end with observations on man, whatever the intermediate steps may be."

The observer may well have to be more patient than the experimenter — awaiting the occurrence of the natural succession of events he desires to study; he may well have to be more imaginative — sensing the correlations that lie below the surface of his observations; and he may well have to be more logical and less dogmatic — avoiding as the evil eye the fallacy of *post hoc ergo propter hoc*, the mistaking of correlation for causation.

Lastly, I quote the words of Professor William Topley,[13] a British worker for whom I had a profound admiration and from whose wisdom I endeavored to learn:

A great part of clinical medicine, and of epidemiology, must still be observation. Nature makes the experiments, and we watch and understand them if we can. No one will deny that we should always aim at planned intervention and closer control. Here, as elsewhere, technique — the way we make our observations and check them — is half the battle; but to force experiment and observation into sharply separated categories is almost as dangerous a heresy as the science and art [of medicine] antithesis. It tends to make the clinician in the ward, the epidemiologist in the field, and the laboratory worker at his bench, think of themselves as doing different things, and bound by different rules. Actually they are all making experiments, some good, some bad. It is more difficult to make a good experiment in the ward than in the laboratory, because conditions are more difficult to control; but there is no other way of gaining knowledge... Controlled observation in the ward or in the field is an essential part of medical science, shading through almost imperceptible stages of increasing intervention into the fully developed experimental technique of the laboratory.

Mr. Winston Churchill, revisiting the Niagara Falls after more than forty years, was asked by a reporter "Do they look the same?" "Well", he is said to have replied, "the principle seems the same." General principles are obstinate things; they do tend to remain the same generation after generation. Yet one element of that sameness — their fundamental importance — perhaps justifies their being brought out into the light of day from time to time and, if one cannot weave fresh clothes, at least in a newly

Vol. 248 No. 24

dyed costume. In accepting the honor of delivering this Cutter Lecture I indeed trusted that that was so. If I was wrong I must comfort myself like that charming character described by Anatole France: like Monsieur Bonnard, I have the satisfaction of believing that, in following my distinguished predecessors, I have at least "utilized to their fullest extent those mediocre faculties with which Nature endowed me."

REFERENCES

1. Sinclair, H. M. Nutritional surveys of population groups. *New Eng. J. Med.* **245**:39-47, 1951.
2. Yule, G. *The Function of Statistical Method in Scientific Investigation.* (Industrial Health Research Board Report.) No. 28. 14 pp. London: His Majesty's Stationery Office, 1924.
3. Greenwood, M. Is statistical method of any value in medical research? *Lancet* **2**:153-158, 1924.
4. Tippett, L. H. C. *Statistics.* 184 pp. London: Oxford University Press, 1943.
5. Lancaster, H. O. Deafness as epidemic disease in Australia: note on census and institutional data. *Brit. M. J.* **2**:1429-1432, 1951.
6. Stocks, P. *Modern Trends in Public Health.* Edited by A. Massey. 591 pp. London: Butterworth, 1949. Chap. XIX.
7. Himsworth, H. P. *The Application of Scientific Methods to Industrial and Service Medicine.* (Medical Research Council.) London: His Majesty's Stationery Office, 1924. P. 109.
8. Hill, A. B. Cited by Himsworth.[7] P. 7.
9. Linklater, E. *Juan in America.* 466 pp. London: Jonathan Cape, 1931.
10. Platt, R. Wisdom is not enough: reflections on art and science of medicine. *Lancet* **2**:977-980, 1952.
11. Garland, J. *New England Journal of Medicine* and Massachusetts Medical Society. *New Eng. J. Med.* **246**:801-806, 1952.
12. Pickering, G. W. Opportunity and universities. *Lancet* **2**:895-898, 1952.
13. Topley, W. W. C. *Authority, Observation and Experiment in Medicine.* 46 pp. London: Cambridge University Press, 1940. P. 40.

I–2.

Jerome Cornfield: Statistical Relationships And Proof In Medicine. American Statistician 1954; 8:19–21.

Jerome Cornfield's "Statistical Relationships and Proof in Medicine" is a contemporary of and fitting complement to Hill's "Observation and Experiment." Here again the (then) controversial smoking-lung cancer relation may be seen as a driving force leading an eminent biostatistician to defend nonexperimental methods. And here again one can see the foreshadowing of issues raised twenty years later in the discussion of Popper's philosophy—this time in the recognition that proof does not exist in empirical science. Cornfield also took care to point out the limitations of experimental randomization, and the consequent importance of considering alternative explanations of results when planning or interpreting *any* study.

QUESTIONS AND ANSWERS

Edited By ERNEST RUBIN

U. S. Department of Commerce
and American University

Statistical Relationships and Proof in Medicine

Within the last two years a formidable controversy has developed as a result of investigations concerning smoking and lung cancer. Statistical data indicate that smokers have a higher incidence of lung cancer than non-smokers. The experience with the smoking—lung cancer controversy suggested the following question: Are there instances in the history of medicine in which a statistical association proved causation or has the proof of a causal relationship in medicine always depended on direct experimentation? I wish to thank Mr. Jerome Cornfield of the Office of Biometry, National Institutes of Health for preparing the following analysis of this question.

There are several preliminary issues raised by the question that need prior discussion. The first, the concept of proof, need not detain us long. Proof has a well-defined meaning in mathematics, but not in empirical science. The truth of a mathematical proposition can be demonstrated; the evidence for an empirical proposition, i.e., a statement in natural science, can be made strong or even overwhelming (despite the apparent impossibility of a satisfactory calculus of evidence). It is doubtful, however, if such propositions can ever be regarded as proved. New evidence (e.g., the discovery of black swans) may cast an entirely different light on a well-established proposition, and in an empirical science, as opposed to mathematics, there are no postulate systems which delimit the kind of new evidence that can be found. If we ask for proof in medicine, or any other empirical science, we may be asking for something that does not exist.

A second issue raised by the question is the exact nature of the distinction between a relationship based upon a statistical association and one based on direct experimentation. We all have a vague feeling that if we can make an event occur, we understand it better than if we simply observe it passively. On analysis this feeling seems to reduce to two propositions like the following: We are initially skeptical of any relationship based upon simple observation because the effects of other possibly important variables are not controlled and may account for the observed association. We are initially impressed by any relationship established by experiment because we feel that the effects of other important variables are controlled and cannot account

for the association. The distinction we feel between a relationship based upon a statistical association and one based upon direct experimentation is thus a distinction between relationships that may be explained by other variables and those that cannot.

Although this statement may formalize our intuitions it is an oversimplification of the actual facts. First, there are cases in which uncontrolled observations can be so analyzed as to eliminate the possibility that extraneous variables account for the observed association. The classical example of this is Snow's demonstration (1) in the middle of the nineteenth century, before the birth of bacteriology, that cholera was transmitted through polluted water. Even the most skeptical critic cannot quarrel with the conclusions drawn from his observations on the clustering of deaths about a particular source of polluted water, the famous Broad Street pump; particularly after his demonstration that mortality from cholera among subscribers of a water company that drew its supply from the Thames River was 14 times as high as that among subscribers of the competing company whose water was sewage-free. The official inquiry which followed agreed that "fecalized drinking-water . . . may breed and convey the poison [of cholera]" although with a caution that is perhaps not peculiar to the Victorian era added, "[so would] fecalized air."[1] Nor do we have to go back 100 years to find examples in which the effects of specific extraneous variables were eliminated from observational material by methods short of direct experimentation. Cross-classification of observations is an obvious, but often surprisingly powerful method of accomplishing this, for some recent examples of which references (3, 4, 5 and 6) may be instructive.

Secondly, our intuitions may be misleading because there is no automatic guarantee in any particular instance that extraneous variables have been controlled by direct experimentation. This may seem to deny the

---

[1] It is not entirely irrelevant to recall at this point the experience of Max von Pettenkofer who, many years later, to prove beyond any doubt that water-borne bacteria did *not* cause cholera, drank, and induced several of his students to drink, a whole glass full of the bacilli. They not only all survived but reported nothing worse than a bellyache (2).

great virtue claimed for randomization, the automatic balancing out among treatment groups of the effects of other variables, whether or not we are aware of their existence. The denial is more apparent than real, however. Consider for example an experiment designed to study the effect of removing an organ, say the thyroid gland, on some biological response, say blood sugar level. We may randomize animals among a control and thyroidectomized group and thus eliminate in the usual probability sense the possibility that any large difference between the two treatments arose from the different characteristics of the animals treated. But we have not eliminated the possible effect of other extraneous variables in which the experimenter is equally interested such as the operation removing the thyroid, or the non-specific effect of thyroidectomy on weight loss. While it is perhaps possible to control these specific variables, for example, sham operation and under feeding the sham operated controls might be regarded as providing such a control (7), randomization by itself is insufficient. We must indicate the specific variables we wish to control and must devise specific experimental procedures to control them.

Having thus argued that there is no difference in kind between the two types of evidence it is of course necessary to add that there is a very important difference in degree. It is a good deal more difficult to control variables in observational than in experimental material, so that the experimental method has unravelled and will continue to unravel mysteries before which uncontrolled observation would be powerless. But there is no difference in principle. There are no such categories as first-class evidence and second-class evidence. There are merely associations, whether observational or experimental that, in a given state of knowledge, can be accounted for in only one way or in several different ways. If the latter, it is our obligation to state what the alternative explanations or variables might be and to see how their effects can be eliminated, while if the former it is equally our obligation to state so. To distinguish between statistical association on the one hand and relationships that are established by experimentation on the other, without any reference to alternative variables that are present in one case but not the other, seems to us to be neither good statistics, good science, nor good philosophy—though it may be good red herring.

If we consider the tobacco-lung cancer question, for example, one possible set of extraneous variables that might explain the higher incidence for smokers are those arising from self-selection. Thus, some small proportion of the population, say 5 percent, might have some special trait (or traits), say high blood levels of certain hormones, which both initiate lung cancer and make the possessors smoke. Of the remaining adult male population, 75 percent smoke for other reasons

and do not develop lung cancer. It is possible to conceive but impossible to conduct an experiment that could settle this question. A large group of adolescents would be allocated at random to different smoking groups, compelled to remain on the assigned smoking schedule, followed for the 30 to 60 years required for lung cancer to develop and the lung cancer incidence computed for each group. This and, as nearly as one can see, only this, would entirely eliminate self-selection as an explanation. Short of this one must rely upon indirect evidence. If self-selection were the complete explanation of the difference, then tobacco smoke would not be a carcinogen for human lung tissue. One might consequently investigate this question by asking is it a carcinogen for any other type of tissue that one can reasonably experiment with, say human or mouse skin? If the answer had been no, this might have been regarded as some type of evidence for the self-selection hypothesis, although no one would regard the evidence as very strong. The recent induction of skin tumors in mice by tobacco tars (8) might similarly be considered evidence against the self-selection hypothesis, but again far from strong. In any event the recent announcement by the Tobacco Industry Research Committee that it would investigate psychological differences between smokers and nonsmokers suggests that we have not heard the last of the self-selection hypothesis. No matter what one's opinion on the plausibility of this as an explanation,[2] the actual investigation of whether specific differences that might arise from self-selection do in fact account for the association could be constructive, even if the results obtained were negative.

This discussion of preliminary issues[3] in one sense also disposes of the main question, but the history of medicine on this point is interesting and a few words may be in order. There are numerous instances that one can cite in which the most important source of medical knowledge on a subject was supplied by statistical associations. Thus, the observation that there is a close inverse association between the amount of natural fluorides in water and the amount of dental caries among children drinking it, has induced numer-

---

[2] It is easy to sympathize with, even if one cannot entirely share the exasperation expressed by Greenwood and Yule on a related point (9). "[The vaccinated group] may all have been vegetarians, or nonsmokers, or red-headed, and all or any of these things may render them less likely to contract cholera; but we do not see why objections which no sensible man would allow to influence him in the ordinary affairs of life should suddenly acquire scientific importance when the question is one of interpreting statistics."

[3] There is one additional preliminary issue that deserves mention. The phrasing of the question suggests that its framer subscribes to the somewhat old-fashioned view that it is either possible or desirable to discuss knowledge without any reference to the possible actions to which it will lead. I have not challenged this view only because I share it.

ous municipalities to add fluorine to their water supply. The resulting decline in the incidence of dental caries in these municipalities may be considered a "direct experimental proof" of the proposition that fluorine inhibits the development of caries, but the fluorine was not added in order to study this question experimentally but rather to bring about a result indicated by the associations. It is true that the results of adding fluorine to the drinking water of experimental animals also pointed in the same direction (10), but as evidence this apparently was not given much weight. Shaw, for example, in his excellent summary of the subject (11) does not even mention the results with experimental animals.

In the study of the effects of therapy the application of modern ideas of experimental design is a very recent development, for an account of which the reader is referred to Hill's very interesting article (12). In recent years there have been several well-conceived experiments to test the efficacy of different preparations, such as gamma globulin, in protecting against the subsequent development of disease. But methods that were established in the past such as vaccination against smallpox, have never received such a carefully controlled experimental test. There are of course dozens of studies to show that individuals who had been voluntarily vaccinated developed less smallpox than others, and that when they did develop it, the outcome was less frequently fatal. But none of these studies ruled out the possibilities of self-selection any more effectively than they are now ruled out in tobacco-lung cancer studies.

In the study of infectious disease there are naturally almost no examples of direct experimental demonstration on humans. Walter Reed's experiments on yellow fever are well known, but it is difficult to find other cases. Perhaps the nearest is the ghastly episode that occurred in Lübeck in 1926, when out of 249 babies accidentally inoculated with enormous numbers of living virulent tubercle bacilli, 76 died (13). If one is willing to overlook the absence of a placebo-inoculated control group, and refrains from asking, "if the bacilli cause tuberculosis, why didn't all the inoculated children develop the disease?", this perhaps is "proof of a causal relationship." (The 173 Lübeck babies who did not die developed only minor lesions and were still free of tuberculosis when last observed 12 years later.)

In short, if we insist on direct experimental demonstration on humans there are many widely held beliefs that must be regarded as without solid foundation. If we believe that vaccination protects against the development of smallpox it is not because there has been a direct experimental demonstration but rather (a) there is a good deal of evidence that is consistent with this hypothesis, and (b) over the course of many

years no evidence has been produced to support any alternative hypothesis. The truth of the matter appears to be that medical knowledge (and, one suspects, many other kinds as well) has always advanced by a combination of many different kinds of observation, some controlled, and some uncontrolled, some directly and some only tangentially relevant to the problems at hand. Although some methods of observation and analysis are clearly to be preferred to others when a choice is possible, there are no magical methods that invariably lead to the right answer. If we cannot specify exactly what has been learned in medicine from the study of statistical associations, we can at least say that we could not have accumulated the knowledge we have without them.[4]

REFERENCES

1. J. Snow, Snow on Cholera, being a reprint of two papers by John Snow, M.D., 1936, The Commonwealth Fund, New York.
2. R. H. Shryock, The Development of Modern Medicine, 1947, Alfred A. Knopf, New York, p. 292.
3. W. E. Heston, M. K. Deringer, I. R. Hughes and J. Cornfield, Interrelation of specific genes, body weight and development of tumors in mice, 1952, *J. National Cancer Institute, 12:* 1141.
4. E. L. Wynder, J. Cornfield, P. D. Schroff, K. R. Doraiswami, A Study of environmental factors in carcinoma of the cervix, 1954, *Amer. J. Obst. and Gyn., 68:* 1016.
5. W. W. Smith, R. Q. Marston, H. J. Ruth and J. Cornfield, Granulocyte count, resistance to experimental infection and spleen homogenate treatment in irradiated mice, 1954, *Amer. J. Physiol., 178:* 288.
6. W. W. Smith, L. Gonshery, I. M. Alderman and J. Cornfield, Effect of granulocyte count and litter on survival of irradiated mice, 1954, *Amer. J. Physiol., 178:* 474.
7. R. O. Scow and J. Cornfield, Effect of thyroidectomy and food intake on oral and intravenous glucose tolerance in rats, 1954, *Amer. J. Physiol., 179:* 39.
8. E. L. Wynder, E. A. Graham, A. B. Croninger, Experimental production of carcinoma with cigarette tar, 1953, *Cancer Res., 13:* 855.
9. M. Greenwood, Epidemics and Crowd Diseases, 1937, Macmillan Co., New York, p. 96.
10. I. Zipkin and F. J. McClure, Inhibitory effect of fluoride on tooth decalcification by citrate and lactate in vivo, 1949, *J. Dental Research, 28:* 151.
11. J. H. Shaw, Should fluorides be added to public water supplies?, 1954, *Scient. Monthly, 79:* 232.
12. A. B. Hill, The Clinical trial, 1952, *New England J. of Med., 247:* 113.
13. R. and J. Dubos, The White Plague, 1952, Little, Brown & Co., Boston, p. 122.
14. A. B. Hill, Observation and experiment, 1953, *New England J. Med. 248:* 995.

---

[4] After completing this answer my attention was called to Hill's Cutler Lecture on Preventive Medicine (14) in which much the same issues that we have covered were also considered—in, however, a more comprehensive, lucid (and reasonable) manner. The reader is enthusiastically referred to it if he is at all interested in pursuing the subject.

I–3.

Austin Bradford Hill: The Environment and Disease: Association or Causation? Proceedings of the Royal Society of Medicine 1965; 58:295–300.

Hill's "The Environment and Disease: Association or Causation" may be a good example of an article that has been read in quotations and paraphrases more often than in its original form. In it, Hill offered a list of nine aspects of an empirical association to consider when deciding whether an association is causal. This was not the first list of "causal criteria" to be offered, but it was perhaps the most popular. It is unfortunate that in the ensuing decades, this list or similar ones have been presented in textbooks as "criteria" for inferring causality of associations, often in such a manner as to imply that all the conditions are necessary. A careful reading of Hill shows that he did not intend to offer a list of necessary conditions; on the contrary, on page 299 he warned against laying down "hard and fast rules of evidence that *must* be obeyed before we accept cause and effect." As noted later [Rothman, 1982], Hill's only real mistake was to say that *none* of his nine aspects could be considered necessary if the association were indeed causal; in fact, temporality (No. 4) is obviously necessary, as cause must precede effect.

Perhaps the most neglected portion of the article (also on page 299) is his comment on the misuse of significance testing by both scientists and statisticians. Despite his warning against equating statistical and scientific significance, I fear that decades later the situation is little better, and so I would give this section special emphasis in any educational setting.

Reference:

Rothman KJ. Causation and causal inference. Chapter 2 in Schottenfeld D and Fraumeni JF, eds. *Cancer Epidemiology and Prevention.* Philadelphia: WB Saunders, 1982.

Meeting January 14 1965

President's Address

The Environment and Disease: Association or Causation?

by Sir Austin Bradford Hill CBE DSC FRCP(hon) FRS
(*Professor Emeritus of Medical Statistics,
University of London*)

Amongst the objects of this newly-founded Section of Occupational Medicine are firstly 'to provide a means, not readily afforded elsewhere, whereby physicians and surgeons with a special knowledge of the relationship between sickness and injury and conditions of work may discuss their problems, not only with each other, but also with colleagues in other fields, by holding joint meetings with other Sections of the Society'; and, secondly, 'to make available information about the physical, chemical and psychological hazards of occupation, and in particular about those that are rare or not easily recognized'.

At this first meeting of the Section and before, with however laudable intentions, we set about instructing our colleagues in other fields, it will be proper to consider a problem fundamental to our own. How in the first place do we detect these relationships between sickness, injury and conditions of work? How do we determine what are physical, chemical and psychological hazards of occupation, and in particular those that are rare and not easily recognized?

There are, of course, instances in which we can reasonably answer these questions from the general body of medical knowledge. A particular, and perhaps extreme, physical environment cannot fail to be harmful; a particular chemical is known to be toxic to man and therefore suspect on the factory floor. Sometimes, alternatively, we may be able to consider what *might* a particular environment do to man, and then see whether such consequences are indeed to be found. But more often than not we have no such guidance, no such means of proceeding; more often than not we are dependent upon our observation and enumeration of defined events for which we then seek antecedents. In other words we see that the event B is associated with the environmental feature A, that, to take a specific example, some form of respiratory illness is associated with a dust in the environment. In what circumstances can we pass from this observed *association* to a verdict of *causation*? Upon what basis should we proceed to do so?

I have no wish, nor the skill, to embark upon a philosophical discussion of the meaning of 'causation'. The 'cause' of illness may be immediate and direct, it may be remote and indirect underlying the observed association. But with the aims of occupational, and almost synonymously preventive, medicine in mind the decisive question is whether the frequency of the undesirable event B will be influenced by a change in the environmental feature A. *How* such a change exerts that influence may call for a great deal of research. However, before deducing 'causation' and taking action we shall not invariably have to sit around awaiting the results of that research. The whole chain may have to be unravelled or a few links may suffice. It will depend upon circumstances.

Disregarding then any such problem in semantics we have this situation. Our observations reveal an association between two variables, perfectly clear-cut and beyond what we would care to attribute to the play of chance. What aspects of that association should we especially consider before deciding that the most likely interpretation of it is causation?

(1) *Strength*. First upon my list I would put the strength of the association. To take a very old example, by comparing the occupations of patients with scrotal cancer with the occupations of patients presenting with other diseases, Percival Pott could reach a correct conclusion because of the *enormous* increase of scrotal cancer in the chimney sweeps. 'Even as late as the second decade of the twentieth century', writes Richard Doll (1964), 'the mortality of chimney sweeps from scrotal cancer was some 200 times that of workers who were not specially exposed to tar or mineral oils and in the eighteenth century the relative difference is likely to have been much greater.'

To take a more modern and more general example upon which I have now reflected for over fifteen years, prospective inquiries into smoking have shown that the death rate from cancer of the lung in cigarette smokers is nine to ten times the rate in non-smokers and the rate in heavy cigarette smokers is twenty to thirty times

296   **Proceedings of the Royal Society of Medicine**   *8*

as great. On the other hand the death rate from coronary thrombosis in smokers is no more than twice, possibly less, the death rate in non-smokers. Though there is good evidence to support causation it is surely much easier in this case to think of some features of life that may go hand-in-hand with smoking – features that might conceivably be the real underlying cause or, at the least, an important contributor, whether it be lack of exercise, nature of diet or other factors. But to explain the pronounced excess in cancer of the lung in any other environmental terms requires some feature of life so intimately linked with cigarette smoking and with the amount of smoking that such a feature should be easily detectable. If we cannot detect it or reasonably infer a specific one, then in such circumstances I think we are reasonably entitled to reject the vague contention of the armchair critic 'you can't prove it, there *may* be such a feature'.

Certainly in this situation I would reject the argument sometimes advanced that what matters is the absolute difference between the death rates of our various groups and not the ratio of one to other. That depends upon what we want to know. If we want to know how many extra deaths from cancer of the lung will take place through smoking (i.e. presuming causation), then obviously we must use the absolute differences between the death rates – 0·07 per 1,000 per year in non-smoking doctors, 0·57 in those smoking 1–14 cigarettes daily, 1·39 for 15–24 cigarettes daily and 2·27 for 25 or more daily. But it does not follow here, or in more specifically occupational problems, that this best measure of the effect upon mortality is also the best measure in relation to ætiology. In this respect the ratios of 8, 20 and 32 to 1 are far more informative. It does not, of course, follow that the differences revealed by ratios are of any practical importance. Maybe they are, maybe they are not; but that is another point altogether.

We may recall John Snow's classic analysis of the opening weeks of the cholera epidemic of 1854 (Snow 1855). The death rate that he recorded in the customers supplied with the grossly polluted water of the Southwark and Vauxhall Company was in truth quite low – 71 deaths in each 10,000 houses. What stands out vividly is the fact that the small rate is 14 times the figure of 5 deaths per 10,000 houses supplied with the sewage-free water of the rival Lambeth Company.

In thus putting emphasis upon the strength of an association we must, nevertheless, look at the obverse of the coin. We must not be too ready to dismiss a cause-and-effect hypothesis merely on

the grounds that the observed association appears to be slight. There are many occasions in medicine when this is in truth so. Relatively few persons harbouring the meningococcus fall sick of meningococcal meningitis. Relatively few persons occupationally exposed to rat's urine contract Weil's disease.

(2) Consistency: Next on my list of features to be specially considered I would place the *consistency* of the observed association. Has it been repeatedly observed by different persons, in different places, circumstances and times?

This requirement may be of special importance for those rare hazards singled out in the Section's terms of reference. With many alert minds at work in industry today many an environmental association may be thrown up. Some of them on the customary tests of statistical significance will appear to be unlikely to be due to chance. Nevertheless whether chance is the explanation or whether a true hazard has been revealed may sometimes be answered only by a repetition of the circumstances and the observations.

Returning to my more general example, the Advisory Committee to the Surgeon-General of the United States Public Health Service found the association of smoking with cancer of the lung in 29 retrospective and 7 prospective inquiries (US Department of Health, Education & Welfare 1964). The lesson here is that broadly the same answer has been reached in quite a wide variety of situations and techniques. In other words we can justifiably infer that the association is not due to some constant error or fallacy that permeates every inquiry. And we have indeed to be on our guard against that.

Take, for instance, an example given by Heady (1958). Patients admitted to hospital for operation for peptic ulcer are questioned about recent domestic anxieties or crises that may have precipitated the acute illness. As controls, patients admitted for operation for a simple hernia are similarly quizzed. But, as Heady points out, the two groups may not be *in pari materia*. If your wife ran off with the lodger last week you still have to take your perforated ulcer to hospital without delay. But with a hernia you might prefer to stay at home for a while – to mourn (or celebrate) the event. No number of exact repetitions would remove or necessarily reveal that fallacy.

We have, therefore, the somewhat paradoxical position that the different results of a different inquiry certainly cannot be held to refute the original evidence; yet the same results from precisely the same form of inquiry will not invariably greatly strengthen the original evidence. I would myself put a good deal of weight upon similar results reached in quite different ways, e.g. prospectively and retrospectively.

Once again looking at the obverse of the coin there will be occasions when repetition is absent or impossible and yet we should not hesitate to draw conclusions. The experience of the nickel refiners of South Wales is an outstanding example. I quote from the Alfred Watson Memorial Lecture that I gave in 1962 to the Institute of Actuaries:

'The population at risk, workers and pensioners, numbered about one thousand. During the ten years 1929 to 1938, sixteen of them had died from cancer of the lung, eleven of them had died from cancer of the nasal sinuses. At the age specific death rates of England and Wales at that time, one might have anticipated one death from cancer of the lung (to compare with the 16), and a fraction of a death from cancer of the nose (to compare with the 11). In all other bodily sites cancer had appeared on the death certificate 11 times and one would have expected it to do so 10–11 times. There had been 67 deaths from all other causes of mortality and over the ten years' period 72 would have been expected at the national death rates. Finally division of the population at risk in relation to their jobs showed that the excess of cancer of the lung and nose had fallen wholly upon the workers employed in the chemical processes.

'More recently my colleague, Dr Richard Doll, has brought this story a stage further. In the nine years 1948 to 1956 there had been, he found, 48 deaths from cancer of the lung and 13 deaths from cancer of the nose. He assessed the numbers expected at normal rates of mortality as, respectively 10 and 0·1.

'In 1923, long before any special hazard had been recognized, certain changes in the refinery took place. No case of cancer of the nose has been observed in any man who first entered the works after that year, and in these men there has been no excess of cancer of the lung. In other words, the excess in both sites is uniquely a feature in men who entered the refinery in, roughly, the first 23 years of the present century.

'No causal agent of these neoplasms has been identified. Until recently no animal experimentation had given any clue or any support to this wholly statistical evidence. Yet I wonder if any of us would hesitate to accept it as proof of a grave industrial hazard?' (Hill 1962).

In relation to my present discussion I know of no parallel investigation. We have (or certainly had) to make up our minds on a unique event; and there is no difficulty in doing so.

(3) *Specificity:* One reason, needless to say, is the specificity of the association, the third characteristic which invariably we must consider. If, as here, the association is limited to specific workers and to particular sites and types of disease and there is no association between the work and other modes of dying, then clearly that is a strong argument in favour of causation.

We must not, however, over-emphasize the importance of the characteristic. Even in my present example there is a cause and effect relationship with two different sites of cancer – the lung and the nose. Milk as a carrier of infection and, in that sense, the cause of disease can produce such a disparate galaxy as scarlet fever, diphtheria, tuberculosis, undulant fever, sore throat, dysentery and typhoid fever. Before the discovery of the underlying factor, the bacterial origin of disease, harm would have been done by pushing too firmly the need for specificity as a necessary feature before convicting the dairy.

Coming to modern times the prospective investigations of smoking and cancer of the lung have been criticized for not showing specificity – in other words the death rate of smokers is higher than the death rate of non-smokers from many causes of death (though in fact the results of Doll & Hill, 1964, do not show that). But here surely one must return to my first characteristic, the strength of the association. If other causes of death are raised 10, 20 or even 50% in smokers whereas cancer of the lung is raised 900–$1,000\%$ we have specificity – a specificity in the magnitude of the association.

We must also keep in mind that diseases may have more than one cause. It has always been possible to acquire a cancer of the scrotum without sweeping chimneys or taking to mule-spinning in Lancashire. One-to-one relationships are not frequent. Indeed I believe that multi-causation is generally more likely than single causation though possibly if we knew all the answers we might get back to a single factor.

In short, if specificity exists we may be able to draw conclusions without hesitation; if it is not apparent, we are not thereby necessarily left sitting irresolutely on the fence.

(4) *Temporality:* My fourth characteristic is the temporal relationship of the association – which is the cart and which the horse? This is a question which might be particularly relevant with diseases of slow development. Does a particular diet lead to disease or do the early stages of the disease lead to those peculiar dietetic habits? Does a

particular occupation or occupational environment promote infection by the tubercle bacillus or are the men and women who select that kind of work more liable to contract tuberculosis whatever the environment – or, indeed, have they already contracted it? This temporal problem may not arise often but it certainly needs to be remembered, particularly with selective factors at work in industry.

(5) *Biological gradient:* Fifthly, if the association is one which can reveal a biological gradient, or dose-response curve, then we should look most carefully for such evidence. For instance, the fact that the death rate from cancer of the lung rises linearly with the number of cigarettes smoked daily, adds a very great deal to the simpler evidence that cigarette smokers have a higher death rate than non-smokers. That comparison would be weakened, though not necessarily destroyed, if it depended upon, say, a much heavier death rate in light smokers and a lower rate in heavier smokers. We should then need to envisage some much more complex relationship to satisfy the cause-and-effect hypothesis. The clear dose-response curve admits of a simple explanation and obviously puts the case in a clearer light.

The same would clearly be true of an alleged dust hazard in industry. The dustier the environment the greater the incidence of disease we would expect to see. Often the difficulty is to secure some satisfactory quantitative measure of the environment which will permit us to explore this dose-response. But we should invariably seek it.

(6) *Plausibility:* It will be helpful if the causation we suspect is biologically plausible. But this is a feature I am convinced we cannot demand. What is biologically plausible depends upon the biological knowledge of the day.

To quote again from my Alfred Watson Memorial Lecture (Hill 1962), there was

'. . . no biological knowledge to support (or to refute) Pott's observation in the 18th century of the excess of cancer in chimney sweeps. It was lack of biological knowledge in the 19th that led a prize essayist writing on the value and the fallacy of statistics to conclude, amongst other "absurd" associations, that "it could be no more ridiculous for the stranger who passed the night in the steerage of an emigrant ship to ascribe the typhus, which he there contracted, to the vermin with which bodies of the sick might be infected". And coming to nearer times, in the 20th century there was no biological knowledge to support the evidence against rubella.'

In short, the association we observe may be one new to science or medicine and we must not dismiss it too light-heartedly as just too odd. As Sherlock Holmes advised Dr Watson, 'when you have eliminated the impossible, whatever remains, *however improbable*, must be the truth.'

(7) *Coherence:* On the other hand the cause-and-effect interpretation of our data should not seriously conflict with the generally known facts of the natural history and biology of the disease – in the expression of the Advisory Committee to the Surgeon-General it should have coherence.

Thus in the discussion of lung cancer the Committee finds its association with cigarette smoking coherent with the temporal rise that has taken place in the two variables over the last generation and with the sex difference in mortality – features that might well apply in an occupational problem. The known urban/rural ratio of lung cancer mortality does not detract from coherence, nor the restriction of the effect to the lung.

Personally, I regard as greatly contributing to coherence the histopathological evidence from the bronchial epithelium of smokers and the isolation from cigarette smoke of factors carcinogenic for the skin of laboratory animals. Nevertheless, while such laboratory evidence can enormously strengthen the hypothesis and, indeed, may determine the actual causative agent, the lack of such evidence cannot nullify the epidemiological observations in man. Arsenic can undoubtedly cause cancer of the skin in man but it has never been possible to demonstrate such an effect on any other animal. In a wider field John Snow's epidemiological observations on the conveyance of cholera by the water from the Broad Street pump would have been put almost beyond dispute if Robert Koch had been then around to isolate the vibrio from the baby's nappies, the well itself and the gentleman in delicate health from Brighton. Yet the fact that Koch's work was to be awaited another thirty years did not really weaken the epidemiological case though it made it more difficult to establish against the criticisms of the day – both just and unjust.

(8) *Experiment:* Occasionally it is possible to appeal to experimental, or semi-experimental, evidence. For example, because of an observed association some preventive action is taken. Does it in fact prevent? The dust in the workshop is reduced, lubricating oils are changed, persons stop smoking cigarettes. Is the frequency of the associated events affected? Here the strongest

support for the causation hypothesis may be revealed.

(9) *Analogy:* In some circumstances it would be fair to judge by analogy. With the effects of thalidomide and rubella before us we would surely be ready to accept slighter but similar evidence with another drug or another viral disease in pregnancy.

Here then are nine different viewpoints from all of which we should study association before we cry causation. What I do not believe – and this has been suggested – is that we can usefully lay down some hard-and-fast rules of evidence that *must* be obeyed before we accept cause and effect. None of my nine viewpoints can bring indisputable evidence for or against the cause-and-effect hypothesis and none can be required as a *sine qua non.* What they can do, with greater or less strength, is to help us to make up our minds on the fundamental question – is there any other way of explaining the set of facts before us, is there any other answer equally, or more, likely than cause and effect?

Tests of Significance
No formal tests of significance can answer those questions. Such tests can, and should, remind us of the effects that the play of chance can create, and they will instruct us in the likely magnitude of those effects. Beyond that they contribute nothing to the 'proof' of our hypothesis.

Nearly forty years ago, amongst the studies of occupational health that I made for the Industrial Health Research Board of the Medical Research Council was one that concerned the workers in the cotton-spinning mills of Lancashire (Hill 1930). The question that I had to answer, by the use of the National Health Insurance records of that time, was this: Do the workers in the cardroom of the spinning mill, who tend the machines that clean the raw cotton, have a sickness experience in any way different from that of other operatives in the same mills who are relatively unexposed to the dust and fibre that were features of the cardroom? The answer was an unqualified 'Yes'. From age 30 to age 60 the cardroom workers suffered over three times as much from respiratory causes of illness whereas from non-respiratory causes their experience was not different from that of the other workers. This pronounced difference with the respiratory causes was derived not from abnormally long periods of sickness but rather from an excessive number of repeated absences from work of the cardroom workers.

All this has rightly passed into the limbo of forgotten things. What interests me today is this: My results were set out for men and women separately and for half a dozen age groups in 36 tables. So there were plenty of sums. Yet I cannot find that anywhere I thought it necessary to use a test of significance. The evidence was so clear-cut, the differences between the groups were mainly so large, the contrast between respiratory and non-respiratory causes of illness so specific, that no formal tests could really contribute anything of value to the argument. So why use them?

Would we think or act that way today? I rather doubt it. Between the two world wars there was a strong case for emphasizing to the clinician and other research workers the importance of not overlooking the effects of the play of chance upon their data. Perhaps too often generalities were based upon two men and a laboratory dog while the treatment of choice was deduced from a difference between two bedfuls of patients and might easily have no true meaning. It was therefore a useful corrective for statisticians to stress, and to teach the need for, tests of significance merely to serve as guides to caution before drawing a conclusion, before inflating the particular to the general.

I wonder whether the pendulum has not swung too far – not only with the attentive pupils but even with the statisticians themselves. To decline to draw conclusions without standard errors can surely be just as silly? Fortunately I believe we have not yet gone so far as our friends in the USA where, I am told, some editors of journals will return an article because tests of significance have not been applied. Yet there are innumerable situations in which they are totally unnecessary – because the difference is grotesquely obvious, because it is negligible, or because, whether it be formally significant or not, it is too small to be of any practical importance. What is worse the glitter of the *t* table diverts attention from the inadequacies of the fare. Only a tithe, and an unknown tithe, of the factory personnel volunteer for some procedure or interview, 20% of patients treated in some particular way are lost to sight, 30% of a randomly-drawn sample are never contacted. The sample may, indeed, be akin to that of the man who, according to Swift, 'had a mind to sell his house and carried a piece of brick in his pocket, which he showed as a pattern to encourage purchasers'. The writer, the editor and the reader are unmoved. The magic formulæ are there.

Of course I exaggerate. Yet too often I suspect we waste a deal of time, we grasp the shadow and lose the substance, we weaken our capacity to interpret data and to take reasonable decisions whatever the value of P. And far too often we deduce 'no difference' from 'no significant difference'. Like fire, the χ^2 test is an excellent servant and a bad master.

The Case for Action
Finally, in passing from association to causation I believe in 'real life' we shall have to consider what flows from that decision. On scientific grounds we should do no such thing. The evidence is there to be judged on its merits and the judgment (in that sense) should be utterly independent of what hangs upon it – or who hangs because of it. But in another and more practical sense we may surely ask what is involved in our decision. In occupational medicine our object is usually to take action. If this be operative cause and that be deleterious effect, then we shall wish to intervene to abolish or reduce death or disease.

While that is a commendable ambition it almost inevitably leads us to introduce differential standards before we convict. Thus on relatively slight evidence we might decide to restrict the use of a drug for early-morning sickness in pregnant women. If we are wrong in deducing causation from association no great harm will be done. The good lady and the pharmaceutical industry will doubtless survive.

On fair evidence we might take action on what appears to be an occupational hazard, e.g. we might change from a probably carcinogenic oil to a non-carcinogenic oil in a limited environment and without too much injustice if we are wrong. But we should need very strong evidence before we made people burn a fuel in their homes that they do not like or stop smoking the cigarettes and eating the fats and sugar that they do like. In asking for very strong evidence I would, however, repeat emphatically that this does not imply crossing every 't', and swords with every critic, before we act.

All scientific work is incomplete – whether it be observational or experimental. All scientific work is liable to be upset or modified by advancing knowledge. That does not confer upon us a freedom to ignore the knowledge we already have, or to postpone the action that it appears to demand at a given time.

Who knows, asked Robert Browning, but the world may end tonight? True, but on available evidence most of us make ready to commute on the 8.30 next day.

REFERENCES
Doll R (1964) In: Medical Surveys and Clinical Trials. Ed. L J Witts. 2nd ed. London; p 333
Doll R & Hill A B (1964) *Brit. med. J.* i, 1399, 1460
Heady J A (1958) *Med. World, Lond.* 89, 305
Hill A B
(1930) Sickness amongst Operatives in Lancashire Spinning Mills. Industrial Health Research Board Report No. 59. HMSO, London
(1962) *J. Inst. Actu.* 88, 178
Snow J (1855) On the Mode of Communication of Cholera. 2nd ed. London (Reprinted 1936, New York)
US Department of Health, Education & Welfare (1964) Smoking and Health. Public Health Service Publication No. 1103. Washington

I–4.

Philip E. Sartwell: "On the Methodology of Investigations of Etiologic Factors in Chronic Disease" – Further Comments. Journal of Chronic Diseases 1960; 11:61–63.

The following paper by Sartwell appeared as a comment on an extended article, "On the Methodology of Investigations of Etiologic Factors in Chronic Diseases," by Yerushalmy and Palmer [1959]. I chose not to include the latter article in this collection because of space limitations and also because the criterion-oriented approach to causal inference favored by Yerushalmy and Palmer was more thoughtfully and influentially put forth by Austin Bradford Hill. Sartwell's response, however, contained elements too good to pass up, as well as comments relevant to Hill's criteria. I refer the reader especially to the delightful anecdote under Sartwell's point 5, and his forceful rejection of the criterion of "specificity of effect."

Reference:

Yerushalmy J, Palmer CE. On the methodology of investigations of etiologic factors in chronic diseases. J Chron Dis 1959; 10:27–40 (with comments by AM Lilienfeld on pages 41–46).

Reprinted from Journal of Chronic Diseases, St. Louis
Vol. 11, No. 1, Pages 61-63, January, 1960
(Copyright © 1960 by The C. V. Mosby Company) (Printed in the U.S.A.)

"ON THE METHODOLOGY OF INVESTIGATIONS OF ETIOLOGIC FACTORS IN CHRONIC DISEASES"—FURTHER COMMENTS

Philip E. Sartwell, M.D.

Baltimore, Md.

From the Department of Epidemiology, Johns Hopkins School of Hygiene and Public Health

(Received for publication Aug. 18, 1959)

YERUSHALMY and Palmer[1] have invited general discussion of their thoughtful article, "On the Methodology of Investigations of Etiologic Factors in Chronic Diseases." I shall not attempt anything as ambitious as a modification of their suggested postulates, although I do not agree with the third statement in their formulation. It may be helpful, however, to enumerate some points which should affect the weight given to epidemiologic evidence for the hypothesis that some environmental factor (E) is an etiologic agent (or vector for the etiologic agent) of a chronic disease.

    1. *The Strength of the Association.*—This quality, mentioned by Lilienfeld[2] in his comments on the article, has two aspects:

    a. How frequently is E found in cases of the disease? Existence of many cases of the disease without E does not invalidate the hypothesis (since the disease may have multiple causes), but it weakens it.

    b. How often does E occur in the absence of the disease? A considerable frequency of E in the general population does not necessarily weaken the hypothesis, because in all diseases of known causation there are accessory factors affecting susceptibility. Our knowledge concerning most of these factors is very meager. To use an analogy from infectious diseases, there are many healthy persons who harbor the meningococcus or poliovirus for every clinical case of meningococcic meningitis or paralytic poliomyelitis.

    2. *Confirmation of the Association by Replication.*—(Studies by different investigators, in different populations.)

    3. *The Quantitative Relationship Between the Amount of E and Frequency of Disease.*—Amount of E may be measured in duration of exposure, in average intensity of exposure, or perhaps best in some integration of these two factors which will give a measure of the total lifetime exposure (for example, the total roentgens of ionizing radiation). Needless to say, since age is a determinant of practically all diseases, adjustment for age effects must be made or spurious conclusions may be drawn.

4. *Chronologic Relationships.*—(Implied in Yerushalmy and Palmer's generalized statement of Koch's postulates and related to the preceding point.) E must precede the disease. But more than this, we may occasionally hope to demonstrate a curve of latent periods, as has been possible in a few instances where a single brief exposure to E is responsible for a disease (as in the occurrence of leukemia in Hiroshima and Nagasaki after the atomic bombings).

Another aspect of this point is the presence of parallelism between the time trends of E and incidence of the disease in the population. This so frequently results from indirect and meaningless association that, if present, it cannot be considered to be materially strengthening the hypothesis; its absence, however, seriously weakens the hypothesis.

It may be charged that points 1 through 4 provide no answer to the logical argument that E may not be the etiologic agent or its vector, but merely a factor indirectly associated with the real, unidentified etiologic agent. But it appears quite logical that the more completely points 1 to 4 are satisfied, the greater the likelihood that we are indeed dealing with agent or vector, because otherwise we should have to postulate an association between E and the true unidentified agent or vector which approaches nearer and nearer to perfect correspondence, in different times, at different places, and in different population groups. This would seem to become more improbable as the association between E and the disease becomes closer.

5. *The Biologic Reasonableness of the Association.*—This point cannot and should not be left out of consideration, but we must be wary of it, for judgments made on this basis are hemmed in by the imperfect knowledge existing at any time. In 1861 Cheever,[3] warning against attaching any significance to "nonsense correlations," wrote, "It could be no more ridiculous for the stranger who passed the night in the steerage of an emigrant ship to ascribe the typhus, which he there contracted, to the vermin with which bodies of the sick might be infested. An adequate cause, one reasonable in itself, must correct the coincidences of simple experience."*

I cannot accept Yerushalmy and Palmer's proposed postulate (No. 3) with respect to specificity of effect. They say, ". . .The suspected characteristic can be said to be specifically related to the disease in question when. . . similar relationships do not exist with a variety of characteristics and with many disease entities when such relationships are not predictable on physiologic, pathologic, experimental, or epidemiologic grounds. In general, the lower the frequency of these other associations, . . . the higher the validity of the causal inference." This statement seems to rest on the assumption that a particular characteristic can induce only a single disease.

Acute gastritis, cirrhosis of the liver, and a form of psychosis are all considered to result directly or indirectly from the ingestion of alcohol in excessive amounts, although it is possible that alcohol acts as a vector, in the broad sense

---

*Dr. Clifford A. Bachrach brought this forceful illustration to the attention of the author.

used by Yerushalmy and Palmer, in one or more of these conditions. The evidence for alcohol as an etiologic agent in cirrhosis (which is mostly clinical rather than epidemiologic) is not weakened by the fact that alcohol is associated with other diseases as well. Application of the specificity concept would also seem to shed doubt on the pathogenicity of atmospheric pollution, which has been linked with several diseases although the evidence to date is limited.

Additional illustrations of what seems to me the fallacy of rejecting the etiologic role of an agent because it is associated with several diseases can readily be thought of in the infectious disease field. For example, streptococci are associated with sore throats, scarlet fever, otitis media, erysipelas, puerperal sepsis, osteomyelitis, and numerous other less common conditions. Use of the specificity concept would lead to rejection of streptococcal causation of each of these conditions, and in fact probably did hinder the acceptance of this organism as the cause of scarlet fever because the relationship was not predictable at the time on the basis of existing biologic grounds.

Perhaps we may be overcautious in rejecting epidemiologic evidence. Snow's[4] demonstration in 1854, referred to repeatedly in discussions of this subject, that cholera was related to the ingestion of polluted water was based on epidemiologic observation rather than experiment. His exposed populations in the Broad Street epidemic and in the South London experience were not selected by random methods. After the publication of his studies, it became accepted that cholera was somehow related to impure water, as some had thought even earlier. His belief that contaminated water contained the specific agent of the disease was, however, not accepted until many years later. Rather, the water was considered as a kind of "predisposing cause" of cholera, among other such predisposing causes. Not until the Hamburg epidemic of 1892, 38 years later, when the cholera vibrio was isolated from the Elbe River, was there conclusive laboratory evidence for Snow's hypothesis. Meanwhile much had been done in England on the basis of Snow's work to improve water supplies. Ought public health authorities in 1854, when the germ theory of disease was in its infancy, to have said, "This is epidemiologic evidence; it is not supported by valid laboratory evidence, and the particular hypothesis that water contains the specific cholera poison is biologically implausible; therefore, we should not act on it"?

REFERENCES

1. Yerushalmy, J., and Palmer, Carroll E.: On the Methodology of Investigations of Etiologic Factors in Chronic Diseases, J. CHRON. DIS. 10:27, 1959.
2. Lilienfeld, Abraham M.: "On the Methodology of Investigations of Etiologic Factors in Chronic Diseases"—Some Comments, J. CHRON. DIS. 10:41, 1959.
3. Cheever, David W.: The Value and Fallacy of Statistics in the Observation of Disease, Boston M. & S. J. 63:449, 1861.
4. Snow, John: On the Mode of Communication of Cholera, London, 1855, John Churchill.

I–5.

Brian MacMahon and Thomas F. Pugh: Causes and Entities of Disease. In *Preventive Medicine*, first edition, edited by Duncan W. Clark and Brian MacMahon Boston: Little, Brown, 1967.

Some of the content of MacMahon and Pugh's "Causes and Entities of Disease" can be found in their textbook *Epidemiology: Principles and Methods* [1970]. Nevertheless, I chose to include the article because the textbook presumably now sees little classroom use, and the points of overlap with the article are "classic" in that they remain valid and forceful today.

I also think the article nicely illustrates the sophistication in thinking about causation that evolved during the post-World War II era, when chronic-disease epidemiology underwent its first major expansion. For example, the section "Diversity of Effects" (p. 16) reflects a more critical attitude toward the criterion of "specificity of effect" engendered by the early debates and findings regarding smoking and health. In addition, the recognition of the circularity inherent in Koch's first postulate (p. 15) exemplifies the break from modes of thought that dominated much of epidemiology in the early 1900's.

The article also forms a bridge between the earlier works of Hill, Cornfield, and Sartwell, and more recent writings on causal inference. For example, MacMahon and Pugh's observation that the labeling of a risk factor as a necessary cause depends on the prevalence of the factor and its cofactors (p. 16) is offered in the practical spirit of Hill but anticipates the discussion of strength of risk factors in the Rothman article of this collection.

Reference:

MacMahon B, Pugh TF. *Epidemiology: Principles and Methods.* Boston: Little, Brown, 1970.

2. *Causes and Entities of Disease*

Brian MacMahon and
Thomas F. Pugh

BASIC to any useful system of disease prevention or therapy is the construction or definition of disease entities. These entities are created by classifying ill persons according to characteristics thought to have relevance in respect to the cause, mechanism, or course of their illnesses. The members of such a group are said to have a specific disease or disease entity.

The arbitrary features in the practice of creating disease entities are frequently not recognized. Ill persons fall into many distinguishable groups—so many that one could readily construct a classificatory scheme that embraced as many disease entities as ill persons and consequently was useless with respect to generalizations of any sort. The disease entities that are in fact recognized have been selected, from the innumerable possibilities that exist, on the basis of usefulness for prevention or treatment or on the basis of medical tradition.

For purposes of prevention, it is most useful to identify as disease entities those in which causal factors are the definitive characteristics. Again, there are innumerable factors in the environment and in genes that are causative of disease. The disease entities created will then vary considerably according to the causal factors that are selected as the basis of classification. The selection is arbitrary and is determined by the utility of the disease entity created or by the priority of discovery of the association of a particular causal factor with a group of ill persons. Significant new knowledge of etiology may bring about major revisions of the boundaries of existing entities. ·

It is evident therefore that concepts of what constitutes a cause of disease and how diseases should be classified for preventive purposes are closely intertwined.

12 / Methods in Preventive Medicine

CONCEPTS OF CAUSE

An appropriate definition of cause is that of J. S. Mill [3]: "The cause, then, philosophically speaking, is the sum total of the conditions positive and negative taken together; the whole of the contingencies of every description, which being realized, the consequent invariably follows." Note that Mill's definition is empiric—given certain conditions, other conditions are observed—and does not require knowledge of the mechanism of the relationship. As Hume [2] earlier remarked: "We are never able, in a single instance, to discover any power or necessary connection, any quality which binds the effect to the cause, and renders the one an infallible consequence of the other. We only find that one does actually, in fact, follow the other."

In terms of Mill's definition, it is evident that the goal of understanding the cause of any disease or event clearly is not attainable. The only practical aim can be the identification of some of the components in the infinite causal web. While it is hopeless to attempt to answer the question "What is the cause of this disease?", it may be possible to obtain an answer to such questions as "What are some of the causal contingencies in this disease?" or "Is this factor a cause of this disease?"

In the last question, the query is whether the factor A is one of the contingencies that in toto constitute Mill's cause of event B. If it is, then A being present and all the other contingencies operative, B will invariably follow.

In practice, it must be determined whether A is one of the causal contingencies of disease B in the absence of knowledge of what the other contingencies are. In the absence of such knowledge, an assumption may be made that the other contingencies are distributed equally between persons who experience A and those who do not. If this is the case, and if A is a cause of B, a higher frequency of B will be found in A persons than in not-A persons, even though B is not found in all A persons. The first requirement in determining that A is a cause of B, then, is that a statistical association exists between A and B.

Not all instances of statistical association are indicative of a causal relationship. That A is a cause of B implies that B would not have occurred in the absence of A, a criterion not met by many statistical associations. For example, both cholera and typhoid fever may depend on poor sewage disposal and thus be statistically associated, but cholera would not be considered a cause of typhoid fever or vice versa.

A statistical association can be defined as causal when there is an association between two categories of events such that alteration of one (the cause) is observed to be followed by a change in the frequency or quality of the other (the effect). If the supposed cause cannot be, or has not been, altered, an association may be classed presumptively as causal when it is believed that, had the cause been altered, the effect would have been changed.

INVESTIGATION FOR CAUSAL RELATIONSHIP

In investigating the possible causal nature of an observed association between two categories of events, an experiment may be designed to determine whether in fact a change in one follows a change in the other. In such an experiment, the subjects are divided at random into two or more groups to ensure that, within the limits of chance variation (which can be estimated), the groups are highly similar. One group is exposed to the suspected factor, and the other is not. Because of the random nature of their selection, it may be assumed that the groups are exposed equally to all other contingencies, and differences in outcome (B) between the groups are judged to be effects of the manipulated factor (A). This model embodies the concept underlying tests applied with increasing frequency to the evaluation of drugs, other therapeutic procedures, and such preventive measures as vaccines and fluoridation of water supplies.

In many instances, random assignment to experimental groups is impracticable, unethical, or undesirable because of medical tradition. Here judgment whether the association is causal becomes difficult, because it must depend on <u>observational</u> data, and the validity of the assumption regarding random distribution of the "other contingencies" is always open to question. Three types of evidence may be brought to bear on the judgment:

1. Strength of the statistical association. The frequency with which two types of events would be expected to occur together by chance within a specified time or geographic distance can be calculated from their separate frequencies. The more frequently the two are in fact observed together, compared with the expected chance frequency, the more probably their association is explained by a causal relationship between them.

2. Time sequence. Instances of the supposed cause should precede instances of the supposed effect.

3. Consistency with existing knowledge. Existing knowledge often suggests that a mechanism linking the proposed cause and effect is conceivable. The existence of a series of known cause-effect associations (A:B, B:C, C:D) would make a proposal of an overall association (A:D) seem not only understandable, but even probable. Existing knowledge may also suggest analogies with currently accepted causal associations that make the causal quality of the one under consideration more reasonable. Thus, there may be considerable resistance to recognition and acceptance of the first example of a new type of factor as a disease-causing agent, but once the first example has been accepted (for example, a microorganism or a genetic element), other agents of the same type are more readily recognized and accepted.

A strong case as to the causal nature of an association can often be built from observational evidence. In the absence of controlled experiment, however, it is possible always to doubt the causal nature of an association and to offer other explanations of the observations. When controlled experiment is not possible, the demand for absolute proof of causation in diseases of human beings is unrealistic. A critical point of view in interpreting observational relationships as causal is prudent, but at some point in the accumulation of evidence, it becomes wiser to accept the causal hypothesis as a basis for action than to continue to debate its validity. Controversy should be limited to discussion of where this point lies, rather than focus on an unrealistic demand for absolute proof of one hypothesis or the other.

NOMENCLATURE AND CLASSIFICATION

A nomenclature is a list of names or designations, with specification as to the characteristics of the things subsumed by the individual designations. A classification is a systematic ordering of such a list. Since the processes of constructing nomenclature and classification are not clearly separable, the latter being dependent on the former, the term classification will be used loosely to include both processes in this discussion.

There are two primary axes of classification of ill persons: manifestational and causal. <u>Manifestational</u> criteria group patients having in common one or more specific manifestations of illness: symptoms, signs, or laboratory determinations. Examples of manifestationally defined illnesses include the common cold, gastric ulcer, and carcinoma of the lung. <u>Causal</u> criteria group patients according to some common prior experience, judged to be of a causal nature. Examples are tuberculosis, avitaminosis, and suicide. All diseases include some manifestational element, if only to the extent that illness is itself a manifestational criterion. Thus, the category of suicide is causally defined, in the sense that it defines a particular cause of death: one's own hand. However, since the state of death is required for inclusion in the category, it is also manifestationally defined. Similarly, the term tuberculosis is usually restricted to persons who, in addition to harboring a causal agent, the tubercle bacillus, also manifest illness.

Originally, disease classification was based primarily on manifestational criteria, and its basis remains predominantly manifestational today. A change to causal criteria is introduced when etiologic factors have been identified as significant and offer promise of major therapeutic or preventive advantage. The recognition of a significant etiologic factor, however, does not necessarily lead to its inclusion in the classification, as it may seem equally useful to continue the manifestational classification. Thus, the identification of cigarette smoking as an important cause of squamous carcinoma of the bronchus has not led to any revision of classification since, for the purpose of therapy—still the dominant purpose of medicine—it is more useful to group patients with bronchial carcinoma together, regardless of cause, than to classify all the different manifestations under "cigarette smoker's disease."

Important to keep in mind is the fact that selection of a particular causal component for the purpose of disease classification depends on its usefulness. The supposition that a chosen component has some more essential relationship to disease than other components may be false, for such a supposition leads occasionally to the misconception that the selected factor is the cause (e.g., that Mycobacterium tuberculosis is the cause of tuberculosis). The importance of this recognition is that existing usefulness does not transcend other possibilities. The desirability of introducing new classifications should be judged by their utility compared to alternate classifications and not on an idea that one classification may be more correct or natural than another.

The pedestrian, struck by an automobile and dying with a ruptured spleen shortly after admission to hospital, is an example. The pathologist may ascribe the death to splenic rupture, the internist to shock, the surgeon to delay in diagnosis in the admitting room. The Registrar of Vital Statistics may be content to assign the death to "Motor vehicle accident involving pedestrian." The highway engineer, in defending his next annual budget, may attribute the death to lack of adequate separation of pedestrian and vehicular traffic, while the engineer responsible for automobile design may count the case among those due to brake failure. Others may point out that the death would not have occurred if the victim had been 25 rather than 65 years old or if his reaction time had not been seriously reduced by alcohol. Each professional observer has selected a different contingency from Mill's causal complex and used it as the basis for his classification. In so doing, he has inferred a special causal relationship of one of the contingencies to the death. Each classification is as valid as another because it is useful for the particular purpose the professional worker had in mind. If the same detail of knowledge existed concerning the etiologic factors in coronary heart disease, no doubt a parallel variety of possible classificatory schemes would exist.

Change from a manifestational to a causal axis of classification may result in a major regrouping of impaired individuals, both in the direction of combining groups with diverse manifestations and of dividing an apparently homogeneous manifestational group. Such a regrouping of impaired persons is exemplified in the one direction by the establishment of syphilis as a disease entity, based on the commonality of interaction with Treponema pallidum. The result is a grouping of such diverse manifestations as chancre, some maculopapular lesions of the skin, aortic insufficiency, and progressive dementia. In the other direction, the term acute yellow atrophy of the liver, no longer in use, once included patients now ascribed to etiologies as separate as toxemia of pregnancy, infectious hepatitis, and various chemical intoxications. Note that the use of the etiologic axis of classification resulted in both instances in entities with diverse manifestations, those of toxemia of pregnancy not being limited to derangement of the liver. Further, no single manifestational entity was reclassified in its entirety to a specific etiologic entity. Thus, not all cases formerly designated as acute yellow atrophy are now classed as infectious hepatitis; nor are all patients with maculopapular rashes, aortic insufficiency, or progressive dementia included with syphilis sufferers.

In this connection, it may be noted that the first of the so-called postulates of Koch[1] is an example of circular reasoning. This postulate states: "The microorganism should be found in all cases of the disease in question, and its distribution should be in accordance with the lesions observed." The circularity of the reasoning lies in the fact that the postulate refers to "the disease in question" as if it had been thought of as an entity before the entire range of effects from the microorganismal element of cause had been identified. In fact, evidence is lacking that the full range of such entities can be recognized before the establishment of causal connection between a disease agent and ill health.

CURRENT CLASSIFICATIONS OF DISEASE ENTITIES

While it is not difficult to understand that the theoretical basis for selection of a classification should be its usefulness, it is very difficult, in selecting a particular classification for general use, to reconcile the different requirements of the many purposes it must serve.

Two disease nomenclatures or classifications are in widespread use in the United States: the Standard Nomenclature [6] published for the American Medical Association and the International Classification of Diseases [8] published by the World Health Organization.

Introduced in 1930 at the initiative of the New York Academy of Medicine, the Standard Nomenclature, now in its fifth edition, is widely used for indexing hospital patients. It "attempts to include every disease which is clinically recognizable." The very exhaustiveness of the nomenclature, however, has led to the situation that a disease of interest to a research worker may be represented by several terms.

The International Classification, in use since 1900, is now in its eighth (1965) revision. Since 1946 the World Health Organization has played a major role in the development and use of this classification, but the successive revisions remain the responsibility of a decennial International Classification Revision Conference representing the user nations. The International Classification is used in the United States and most other countries primarily for the preparation of national statistics on causes of death. Since it is less exhaustive than the Standard Nomenclature and contains many such residual categories as "Injuries of other and unspecified nature," it has been considered unsuitable for clinical use.

An adaptation of the International Classification [4], prepared under the direction of the U.S. National Center for Health Statistics, supplies sufficient specificity for clinical purposes and simultaneously retains the greater statistical simplicity of the parent classification. The adaptation is expected to supersede the Standard Nomenclature in hospital practice.

---

[1]A series of three criteria used by Koch in demonstrating the pathogenicity of M. tuberculosis and referred to as Koch's postulates by later microbiologists. They are itemized by Topley and Wilson [7].

16 / Methods in Preventive Medicine

DIVERSITY OF EFFECTS

Skepticism as to the existence of causal association has been expressed when a proposed cause has been found to be statistically associated with more than one established manifestational entity [5, 9]. For example, the fact that cigarette smoking is associated not only with bronchial cancer but also with chronic bronchitis, coronary heart disease, and even bladder cancer and other diseases has been put forward as an argument that the association with carcinoma of the bronchus is not a causal one, since no cause, it is claimed, should have so many different effects [1]. The assumption that traditional schemes of classifying diseased people, based on manifestational criteria, should be congruent with schemes based on etiology stultifies or delays reconceptualizations that may have both preventive and therapeutic usefulness.

No doubt there is a tendency toward clustering of specific clinical features and other manifestations among patients afflicted with a particular cause of disease, but this by no means amounts to complete correspondence of manifestational and causal groupings. Patients with tuberculosis, for example, include those with a wide variety of manifestations: persons with affections of the bones, lungs, meninges, and skin. Many of these persons would never have been thought of as belonging with others who are currently their nosologic companions except for the presence of M. tuberculosis in their lesions. At the same time other causes (e.g., Histoplasma capsulatum) produce similar polymorphous manifestations often indistinguishable from those "caused" by M. tuberculosis.

One does find diseases in which there is very high association of a particular cause with a particular effect. For example, in certain genetically determined errors of metabolism, a series of mutations of specific single genes is associated with a corresponding series of single enzyme deficiencies that become manifest in quite specific biochemical abnormalities, such as the inability to metabolize phenylalanine. Note that even here the specificity results in part from the arbitrary selection of cause, for the causes responsible for the original genetic mutation in a series of cases of phenylketonuria may be quite varied. Further, a group of patients having an identical enzyme deficiency may show quite varied degrees of mental defect and even include persons with average intelligence. Similarly, there is probably a close, although not complete, correlation between patients defined because of their having a first exposure to measles virus and those defined by having clinical measles, as well as between the members of a group defined because of having been bitten by a rabid animal and those later having clinical rabies.

These examples may suggest that certain factors can be regarded as the <u>necessary</u> cause of particular diseases, with other causal factors relegated to subsidiary or contributory roles. In fact, however, "necessary" causes are necessary only by definition; for example, M. tuberculosis is the necessary cause of tuberculosis, as automobiles are of automobile accidents. A specific genetic deficiency may be thought of as the necessary cause of phenylketonuria, but, in a society in which all were homozygous for the phenylketonuria gene and diets varied in their phenylalanine content, it would be more useful to think of the disease as determined environmentally—by phenylalanine in the diet—and to regard this as the essential factor. The necessary cause is the chosen cause.

In contrast to the above examples, the majority of causal agents that are chosen as criteria for constructing disease entities are associated with a great diversity of clinical, pathological, and biochemical patterns. These patterns often have not been considered part of "one" disease until they have been found to be regularly associated with the chosen agent. Causal agents showing wide variation in their effects from person to person include M. tuberculosis, T. pallidum, alcohol, poverty, the automobile, and "one's own hand."

Past experience, then, suggests that arrangements of ill persons by their manifestations may identify groups that have at least some degree of homogeneity with respect to causal factors and that at least form a useful basis for investigation of cause. Nevertheless, causal factors of disease, when identified, not uncommonly have effects that cross the boundaries of adjacent manifestational groups. In so doing, they produce new groupings of ill persons, some of which alarm nosologists who use tradition as their guiding principle.

CAUSATION AND PREVENTION

Not all demonstrated causal associations are useful bases for preventive measures. This limitation is exemplified by the following considerations:

1. The cause must be amenable to manipulation. Thus, the identification of viral agents in human cancer does not offer the prospect of as rapid a development of preventive measures as might be expected from the identification of microbiological agents in other categories of disease, since special problems are involved in the production of vaccines. As another example, practical measures for preventing genetic damage have not yet been developed.

2. Manipulation of the causal factor must be acceptable. Alcohol, the cigarette, and the automobile are each responsible for an enormous burden of mortality and morbidity in present-day society, but society seems unwilling to give up the benefits associated with them. Lack of acceptability may depend on factors quite unrelated to health.

3. Almost any interference with the existing ecological balance will have effects on health other than those intended or desired. While the "great sanitary awakening" at the turn of this century did rid the Western world of cholera, typhoid, and a great many other diseases, it may also have fostered poliomyelitis and possibly other diseases against which the population was formerly protected because of its unsanitary living conditions and consequent early immunization. Measures such as routine chest x-ray seem imperative under certain conditions and contraindicated under others. The extent of the side effects of preventive measures usually is not known at the time they are introduced. Therefore, periodic surveillance and evaluation of the total effects of such measures are required.

Realization that the directness of a causal association is not necessarily related to its utility for prevention is also important. Directness of causal association is a relative term, dependent on the current state of knowledge of the mechanism of a particular association. Swamps are causally associated with malaria. When this association was found to be explainable because mosquitoes breed in swamps, the association of malaria with mosquitoes was then considered the direct one, and the association with swamps indirect. With the discovery of the malaria parasite, the association with the parasite was considered direct and that with mosquitoes indirect. No doubt there are presently unknown components of the parasite that, when determined, will be considered the more direct causes of malaria ("swamp fever") than the whole parasite.

The more direct the association, the more specific the preventive measure is likely to be and the fewer the anticipated side effects. Thus vaccines, directed specifically against certain infectious agents, tend to produce less ecological disturbance than measures based on indirect aspects of the disease mechanism, for example, sanitary measures. Nevertheless, associations that are recognized as

18 / Methods in Preventive Medicine

being indirect can form the basis of effective preventive measures, either because other more direct associations are not known or because manipulation of the more direct associations is impracticable or inconvenient. The drainage of swamps is still a useful preventive measure against malaria, and the control of cholera in the Western world depends on general sanitary measures rather than immunization.

Knowledge of causal associations that do not offer preventive possibilities, either because from a practical point of view the cause is unalterable or because the side effects are unacceptable, is nevertheless important. Such knowledge aids the study of other potentially causal associations, some of which may be alterable. For example, knowledge of genetic determinants of a disease can facilitate identification of environmental factors involved in its occurrence or severity.

REFERENCES

1. Berkson, J. Smoking and lung cancer: some observations on two recent reports. J. Amer. Statist. Ass. 53:28, 1958.
2. Hume, D. Treatise of Human Nature. (1739.) Selby-Bigge, L. A. (Ed.). Oxford: Clarendon Press, 1896.
3. Mill, J. S. A System of Logic, Ratiocinative and Inductive. (5th Ed.) London: Parker, Son and Bowin, 1862.
4. National Center for Health Statistics. International Classification of Diseases, Adapted for Indexing Hospital Records by Diseases and Operations. Vols. 1 and 2. (Revised Ed.) Pub. Health Service Publ. 719, Washington: Govt. Printing Office, 1962.
5. Sartwell, P. E. On the methodology of investigations of etiologic factors in chronic diseases. Further comments. J. Chronic Dis. 11:61, 1960.
6. Thompson, E. T., and Hayden, A. C. (Eds.). Standard Nomenclature of Diseases and Operations. (5th Ed.) New York: McGraw-Hill (for the American Medical Association), 1961.
7. Topley, W. W. C., and Wilson, G. S. The Principles of Bacteriology and Immunity. (2nd Ed.) Baltimore: William Wood, 1936.
8. World Health Organization. Manual of the International Statistical Classification of Diseases, Injuries, and Causes of Death. Vols. 1 and 2. 7th (1955) Revision. Geneva: World Health Organization, 1957. (The eighth revision was in process in 1966.)
9. Yerushalmy, J., and Palmer, C. E. On the methodology of investigations of etiologic factors in chronic diseases. J. Chronic Dis. 10:27, 1959.

ADDITIONAL READING

Hempel, C. G. Introduction to problems of taxonomy. In Zubin, J. (Ed.), Field Studies in the Mental Disorders. New York: Grune & Stratton, 1961.
Lorr, M., Klett, C. J., and McNair, D. M. Syndromes of Psychosis. New York: Macmillan, 1963.
MacMahon, B., Pugh, T. F., and Ipsen, J. Epidemiologic Methods. Boston: Little, Brown, 1960. Chaps. 2 and 3.
Nowell-Smith, P. H. Causality. In Encyclopaedia Britannica. Chicago: Encyclopaedia Britannica, 1965.

I-6.

Olli Miettinen: Confounding and Effect-Modification.
American Journal of Epidemiology 1974; 100:350–353.

Miettinen's "Confounding and Effect-Modification" is noteworthy for introducing what may be Miettinen's most widely used neologism, "effect modification," and for carefully distinguishing the concept from confounding. The quantitative aspects of this distinction were appreciated by Simpson nearly a quarter of a century previously (see his article in Part II), but a detailed consideration of the causal aspects of these phenomena was not given until Miettinen.

The article was written in response to a brief note by Fisher and Patil [1974], which was in turn inspired by an earlier article by Miettinen. The earlier articles were concerned with issues far afield from effect modification and so are not reproduced here. But it is Miettinen's criteria for confounding and his definition of the term "effect modification" that need to be put in an historical perspective.

Among the criteria for confounding by a covariate (p. 351), items 1–3 are now generally employed, and indeed are often used as a definition of a confounder (i.e., a covariate, predictive of illness among the unexposed and associated with exposure, but not an intermediate variable) (see, e.g., Schlesselman [1982]). Item 4 has not, however, held up under scrutiny: a covariate whose apparent relation to exposure or illness is solely the result of measurement error need not be a confounder [Greenland and Robins, 1985]. And item 5 has been criticized and abandoned by Miettinen himself [Miettinen and Cook, 1981]: among other things, absence of a covariate-illness relation in the data at hand need not imply absence of confounding by the covariate.

With regard to "effect modification"—variation in the chosen effect parameter across levels of a covariate—the term seems somewhat ambiguous, for it suggests a changing biologic process. In fact, as Miettinen notes in point 3 on page 352, when effects are present, presence or absence of effect modification depends on the measure of effect one uses, even if the biological mechanism that produces the effect is invariant. Effect modification is thus no more than a special type of statistical interaction, and should not be confused with biological interaction or "synergy." Given this, a more precise term for the phenomenon would be "effect-measure modification."

One minor technical note: the "Zelen test" of uniformity of the odds ratio, given by Miettinen on page 352, has since been shown to be invalid [Halperin et al., 1977]; for valid tests see, e.g., Schlesselman [1982], or Rothman [1986].

References:

Fisher L, Patil K. Matching and unrelatedness. Am J Epidemiol 1974; 100:347–349.

Greenland S, Robins JM. Confounding and misclassification. Am J Epidemiol 1985; 122:495–506.

Halperin M, Ware JH, Byar DP, et al. Testing for interaction in an I × J × K contingency table. Biometrika 1977; 64:271–275.

Miettinen OS, Cook EF. Confounding: essence and detection. Am J Epidemiol 1981; 114:593–603.

Rothman KJ. *Modern Epidemiology*. Boston: Little, Brown, 1986.

Schlesselman JJ. *Case-control Studies: Design, Conduct, Analysis*. New York: Oxford University Press, 1982.

AMERICAN JOURNAL OF EPIDEMIOLOGY
Copyright © 1974 by The Johns Hopkins University

Vol. 100, No. 5
Printed in U.S.A.

CONFOUNDING AND EFFECT-MODIFICATION

OLLI MIETTINEN[1]

The preceding commentary by Fisher and Patil (1) deals with criteria for a confounding factor and with the distinction between confounding and effect-modification. I take the authors and Editor up on their kind invitation to comment, and I expand on the subtleties of both confounding and effect-modification.

CONFOUNDING: DETAILS FOR CRITERIA

Conditionality on other controlled factors

Fisher and Patil note that two or more factors might jointly constitute a confounder even though each of them singly is devoid of the confounding property. They conclude that the basic criteria for a confounding factor—"relatedness" to both the exposure and the illness at issue (2)—must refer to relationships *conditional* upon all other factors that are considered for control, and they advise efforts to evaluate these conditional associations *instead* of unconditional ones to enhance the detection of confounding.

The formal conclusion reached by Fisher and Patil is, I believe, familiar to epidemiologists: We are aware that the need to control a given factor depends ultimately on its characteristics (relatedness to the exposure and the illness), conditional on whatever other factors are controlled (by restriction, matching, stratification or modelling). This is not only widely recognized but also quite routinely applied in decisions about the need to control.

On the other hand, the practical advice given by Fisher and Patil differs from that already implicit in epidemiologic decision-making. According to these authors one

[1] Department of Epidemiology, School of Public Health, Harvard University, Boston, Mass. 02115.

Supported by grants 5 P01 CA 06373 HE 10436 from the National Institutes of Health.

should not exclude a potential confounding factor from further consideration if it fails to meet the simple (unconditional) criteria. However, epidemiologists in general seem rather content to do just that inasmuch as it seems customary to confine the consideration of conditional relationships to factors for which the simple ones do indicate confounding. In other words, whereas Fisher and Patil advocate *routine* consideration of the conditional relationships with the aim of *detecting* confounding that might otherwise be missed, the prevailing tendency is for *selective* use of the conditional criteria with the aim of *excluding* from control a factor which superficially would appear to be a confounder.

Is there, then, a need for a change in epidemiologic research practice as to the use of simple and conditional criteria for confounding? I believe not. Fisher and Patil are, or course, formally correct even in their procedural advocacy. However, I believe that to pursue routinely the conditional relationships is a policy whose productiveness is much too low to justify the added efforts and complexities relative to the prevailing approach of first "screening" on the basis of unconditional criteria. Rarely is adequate information about the conditional relationships even available, as Fisher and Patil point out; and when it is, the conditional criteria only very exceptionally bring out the confounding property where it was not apparent in terms of the simple relationships. On the other hand, the conditional view is often helpful, even without data, in disposing of a potential confounder. As an example of the latter, when controlling "family" or "neighborhood" through matching, the control of, say, income would be irrelevant even if it were unconditionally associated with both the exposure and the illness.

Meaning of "relatedness"

Fisher and Patil imply that "relatedness" in each of the two criteria for a confounding factor means statistical dependence, but they give no details. Several specifications are worthy of note:

1) The relatedness to the exposure should not be simply a reflection of the exposure influencing the potential confounder. In such a case the factor at issue could be a link in one causal path from the exposure to the illness, and its control would serve only to block the manifestation of this path.

2) The relatedness to the illness must be strictly predictive, i.e., a confounding factor is necessarily a risk indicator for the illness. In fact, in the strictest sense, a confounding factor has a causal connection to the illness. However, since it is generally infeasible to control all causal risk indicators with the confounding property, it is necessary to control them indirectly through their correlates—noncausal risk indicators that are associated with the exposure; by the same token, it is reasonable to regard the latter as actual confounders rather than simply as correlates thereof.

3) The relatedness to the illness must obtain even without mediation by the exposure, i.e., it should not simply reflect association with exposure and the "effect" of the latter. More specifically, the risk indicator status should obtain even "on the null hypothesis" or, equivalently, among the nonexposed. (Risk indicator status among the exposed could result from effect-modification by the potential confounder.)

4) The relationship may be spurious—results of differential biases of selection and/or differential errors of observation over the factor at issue. Thus, a true confounding factor (social class, say) may simply *appear* to be associated with the exposure (intrauterine x-ray exposure, say)

as a result of variations according to this factor in the accessibility to subjects or their records or in errors of information about the exposure; and the factor may be simply an *ostensible* risk indicator because of differential errors in case detection, depending on the category of the factor.

5) Both relationships must obtain in the data of the study at issue. When deciding upon control in the selection of subjects (restriction of range, matching in selecting control subjects), one must, of course, rely on *a priori* information about the outlook —in the absence of control—for the appearance of relationships in the data, and statistical inference might be involved in this (1). On the other hand, in the data-analysis stage the decision about possible control (exclusion of categories, stratification, model fitting) is *not* to be based on statistical inference about (significance testing of) the pertinent associations. In both stages the decisions are to be based on quantitation of the distortive impact of the factor in the absence of co_ntrol. Formal estimation of this may be feasible (3).

EFFECT-MODIFICATION
First principles

Fisher and Patil point out that the magnitude of the "effect"—the parameter for association conditional on controlled confounders—may vary among categories of some factor, and that this factor need not be a confounder of the association. They go no further into the principles of this phenomenon. For placing their note in its proper perspective, it is necessary to appreciate some basic principles of effect-modification:

1) All causally/preventively insufficient exposures have extremely powerful effect-modifiers, which render the effects either total or nonexistent, i.e., which make the exposure causally/preventively either sufficient or inoperative. This may be deduced from the facts that a given illness always results from a sufficient cause, and that the

presence/absence of a given insufficient cause/preventive is a necessary part of some of these sufficient ones; where it is, it is (necessary and) sufficient, whereas otherwise it has no effect at all.

2) All intermediate effect-modification results from differential (latent) weightings of the total and zero effects among the categories of the factor at issue. Since the weights are nothing but relative frequencies of the regions of causal/preventive (sufficiency and) necessity of the exposure at issue, an intermediate effect-modifier need not be a risk indicator conditional on exposure or nonexposure. By the same token, it need not be a confounder (cf. specification no. 3 for "relatedness").

3) All risk indicators, conditional on exposure or nonexposure, modify at least one of the two common epidemiologic measures of effect—risk difference or risk ratio (minus one). Thus, the common assumption of uniformity of risk ratio over a confounder is tantamount to the assumption that, over the range of the confounder, (the absolute value of) risk difference is proportional to the risk of the nonexposed.

Appreciation in data analysis

Fisher and Patil point out, without elaboration, that data analysis without regard for effect-modification can be of suboptimal sensitivity in the detection of the very existence of the association and incomplete in the estimation of its magnitude.

At the same time, routine approaches in epidemiologic data analysis are generally oblivious to possible effect-modification: Common significance tests—the McNemar test (4) and its extension (5) for matched series as well as the more general Mantel-Haenszel test (6) for (matched and) unmatched series—do not provide for nonuniformity of effect. They are, in fact, optimal in the very case where the favorite parameter, risk ratio (or, more accurately, the "odds ratio"), is uniform over the matching categories or the strata of analysis (7). Similarly, common procedures for estimat-

ing this parameter either presuppose uniformity over the matching categories (8) or strata of analysis (9), or they suppress the nonuniformity through "summarization" (6) or standardization (10).

The prevailing habits in significance-testing (for the main null hypothesis of no association conditional on the controlled confounders) cannot be blamed on epidemiologists. For, seemingly no test is known which, by virtue of allowing for nonuniformity of the "odds ratio", would in general tend to be more powerful than the Mantel-Haenszel test (6) or its derivatives (4, 5).

On the other hand, the common failure to look for, and quantify, modification of risk ratio ("odds ratio") is not readily justifiable. As long as the numbers of subjects are sufficient in the categories of the potential modifier, uniformity of this parameter may be tested—against an unspecific alternative—by the use of the statistic $\chi^2 (J - 1) = \Sigma_1 [\chi^2 (1)]_j - \chi^2 (1)$, where $\chi^2 (1)$ is the usual overall chi-square computed without regard for nonuniformity (4-6), and where $[\chi^2 (1)]_j$ is the same statistic computed for the jth one of the J categories of the potential modifier (cf. Zelen (11)). More sensitive testing may also be feasible using an appropriate model for the risk ratio as a function of the modifying factor.

If might seem that the ideal framework for the evaluation of possible modifiers of the "odds ratio" is the "log-linear" model (12), with parameters for interaction between the exposure and other factors interpreted as measures of modification. Thus, if the exposure, coded as 0 for absent and 1 for present, were to have the estimated "main effect" of b_e and "interaction effect" b_{ea} with age (A) but none with other factors in the model, then the age-function of the "odds ratio" might be thought to be exp $(b_e + b_{ea}A)$. I believe that this would be wrong in the usual situation where the model involves other age-related factors (as confounders). After all, when deprived of its correlates (by "keeping them fixed" through the model), "age" becomes a hollow concept, a biologically meaningless number. This pitfall of model interpretation tends to apply, though less strikingly, to sex and many other factors as well, and the problem is not specific to the "log-linear" model but characteristic of multivariate analysis in general.

The solution to this problem of model interpretation is to be sought, I believe, from an appropriate choice of the effect parameter. It seems to me that, in ratio terms, the appropriate parameter is the "standardized morbidity/mortality ratio" for the exposed relative to the nonexposed, evaluated separately within each category of the potential modifier. The standard would vary among the categories (10), but the ratios (minus one) would express the varying "effects", without confounding by the "standardized" factors, for the varying kinds of exposed people in the different categories of the potential modifier. The confounders would thus be controlled as confounders but not as determinants of effect-modification attributed to another factor.

SUMMARY

Confounding and effect-modification —both very central to epidemiologic thinking and research on causality—are closely related but distinctly separate concepts and phenomena. Both of them involve considerable subleties, with implications for problem conceptualization, study design, data analysis and inference. Some of these subtleties and their implications may warrant greater appreciation in the practice of epidemiologic research, while others require further conceptual development.

REFERENCES

1. Fisher L, Patil K: Matching and unrelatedness. Am J Epidemiol 100:347–349, 1974
2. Miettinen OS: Matching and design efficiency in retrospective studies. Am J Epidemiol 91:111–118, 1970
3. Miettinen OS: Components of the crude risk ratio. Am J Epidemiol 96:168–172, 1972
4. McNemar Q: Note on the sampling error of the difference between correlated proportions or percentages. Psychometrika 12:153–157, 1947
5. Miettinen OS: Individual matching with multiple controls in the case of all-or-none responses. Biometrics 25:339–355, 1969
6. Mantel N, Haenszel W: Statistical aspects of the analysis of data from retrospective studies of disease. J Natl Cancer Inst 22:719–748, 1959
7. Birch MW: The detection of partial association. I: The 2 × 2 case. J Roy Statist Soc B 26:313–324, 1964
8. Miettinen OS: Estimation of relative risk from individually matched series. Biometrics 26:75–86, 1970
9. Gart J: The comparison of proportions: a review of significance tests, confidence intervals and adjustments for stratification. Rev Internatl Statist Inst 39:148–169, 1971
10. Miettinen OS: Standardization of risk ratios. Am J Epidemiol 96:383–388, 1973
11. Zelen M: The analysis of several 2 × 2 contingency tables. Biometrika 58:129–137, 1971
12. Worcester J: The relative odds in the 2^3 contingency table. Am J Epidemiol 93:145–149, 1971

I-7.

Kenneth J. Rothman: Causes.
American Journal of Epidemiology 1976; 104:587–592.

Rothman's "Causes" is an exceptionally lucid outline of a point of view regarding causation that has come to be known as the "sufficient/component cause theory." While the theory is a clear descendant of ideas in earlier works (such as MacMahon and Pugh's), it was Rothman who first presented a general schematic form for deducing the relationships between the occurrence of component causes and epidemiologic measures of effect. This schematic form, illustrated in Figure 1 of the paper, allows one to visualize (and thus make precise) the meaning of terms such as "synergy" (which, under the theory, becomes co-participation in a sufficient cause).

I do have one semantic criticism of the paper: At the start of the "synergy" section, Rothman equated "synergy" with "effect modification." It is clear to me, however, that in Miettinen's original use of the term, and much of the usage since, "effect modification" means only "differing values of the effect measure at different levels of another variate," to quote from the introduction of Rothman's paper. As Rothman noted, this implies that the effect modification depends on the scale of measurement. It follows then that "effect modification" cannot in general correspond to "synergy" or co-participation in a sufficient cause, although, as Rothman was aware, certain types of modification of the risk difference would imply the presence of synergistic interactions. More importantly, "effect modification" as defined is a property of events in *populations*, whereas "synergy" is a property of events in *individuals* [Miettinen, 1982]. Perhaps all this only points out again that "effect modification" was a poor term to choose for the phenomenon of effect-measure variation across populations, since it evokes the concept of synergy.

Reference:
Miettinen OS. Causal and preventive interdependence: elementary principles. Scand J Work Env Hlth 1982; 8:159–168.

AMERICAN JOURNAL OF EPIDEMIOLOGY
Copyright © 1976 by The Johns Hopkins University School of Hygiene and Public Health

Vol. 104, No. 6
Printed in U.S.A.

CAUSES

KENNETH J. ROTHMAN

The conceptual framework for causes presented here is intended neither as a review nor an expansion of knowledge, but rather as a viewpoint which bridges the gap between metaphysical notions of cause and basic epidemiologic parameters. The focus, then, is neither metaphysics nor epidemiology, but the gulf between them. In the same spirit as recent discussion on these pages about definitions of basic epidemiologic terms such as *rate* (1), common agreement on the conceptual interrelationship of causes may facilitate communication about causes of illness.

A strong motivation for presenting this scheme is the often-heard confusion of two important but distinct epidemiologic issues: confounding and effect modification. These two properties of variable have different areas of relevance (2). The confounding property is not an intrinsic characteristic of any variable. Confounding, defined as distortion in an effect measure introduced by an extraneous variate, occurs only in the context of a particular study, and the same variable which confounds in one study may not confound the same association in another study setting.

Department of Epidemiology, Harvard School of Public Health, 677 Huntington Avenue, Boston, MA 02115.

In fact, the principles of good study design may call for preventing a potentially confounding variable from being confounding —for example, by matching in the selection of subjects. On the other hand, effect modification, defined as differing values of the effect measure at different levels of another variate, is an inherent characteristic of the relationship between two causes of an illness (effect). This relationship is not governed by the particulars of any study; it is an unalterable fact of nature. To be sure, the magnitude of effect modification depends on the scale of measurement of the effect—for example, a risk ratio which is constant over age generally implies a risk difference which changes with age. But it has been proposed that the risk difference scale is the appropriate scale for assessing effect modification, other scales representing metameters of the risk difference which distort to varying degrees the assessment of effect modification (3). Effect modifiers may or may not be confounders in a given study, or they may confound in some studies but not in others. Conversely, confounders may or may not be effect modifiers. The following discussion presents a scheme for the interrelationship of causes which may provide a useful way for thinking about effect modification as a description of nature.

588   KENNETH J. ROTHMAN

TYPES OF CAUSES

A *cause* is an act or event or a state of nature which initiates or permits, alone or in conjunction with other causes, a sequence of events resulting in an *effect*. A cause which inevitably produces the effect is *sufficient*. The inevitability of disease after a sufficient cause calls for qualification: disease usually requires time to become manifest, and during this gestation, while disease may no longer be preventable, it might be fortuitously cured, or death might intervene.

Common usage makes no distinction between that constellation of phenomena which constitutes a sufficient cause and the components of the constellation which are likewise referred to as "causes". Another qualification for sufficient causes is restriction to the minimum number of required component causes; this implies that the lack of any component cause renders the remaining component causes insufficient. Thus, measles virus is referred to as the cause of measles, whereas a sufficient cause for contracting measles involves lack of immunity to measles virus and possibly other factors in addition to exposure to measles virus. The term *cause*, then, does not specify whether the reference is to a sufficient cause or to a component of a sufficient cause.

Most causes that are of interest in the health field are components of sufficient causes, but are not sufficient in themselves. Drinking contaminated water is not sufficient to produce cholera, and smoking is not sufficient to produce lung cancer, but both of these are components of sufficient causes. Identification of all the components of a given sufficient cause is unnecessary for prevention, in that blocking the causal role of but one component of a sufficient cause renders the joint action of the other components insufficient, and prevents the effect. Even without being able to identify the other components of the sufficient cause for lung cancer, of which smoking is one component, it is possible to prevent those cases of lung cancer which would result from that sufficient cause by removing smoking from the constellation of components.

A specific effect may result from a variety of different sufficient causes. The different constellations of component causes which produce the effect may or may not have common elements. If there exists a component cause which is a member of every sufficient cause, such a component is termed a *necessary* cause. Necessary causes are often identifiable as part of the definition of effect. For example, the possession of a vermiform appendix is necessary for appendicitis, and infection with the tubercle bacillus is a necessary cause for tuberculosis. Though sometimes devoid of useful significance, a necessary cause can be a useful component cause to identify. Whereas many different component causes have been identified for several types of cancer, the hope exists for identification of a final common pathway representing a necessary cause for cancer of all types.

Figure 1 is a schematic illustration of the causal components of a disease. The disease (effect) has three sufficient causal complexes, each having five component causes. In this scheme "A" is a necessary cause, since it appears as a member of each sufficient cause. On the other hand, the component causes "B", "C" and "F", which each appear in more than one sufficient cause, are not necessary causes, because they fail to appear in all three sufficient causes.

ETIOLOGIC FRACTION

Causal research of disease focuses on components of sufficient causes, whether necessary or not. The public health importance of a component cause of disease in a particular population is determined by the fraction of the disease (the effect) which results from the sufficient causes(s) to which the component cause belongs. The epidemiologic parameter *etiologic fraction*

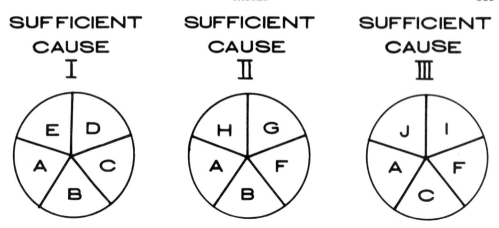

FIGURE 1. Conceptual scheme for the causes of a hypothetical disease.

(4) (population attributable risk) measures this dimension of a cause-effect relationship. Each component of a sufficient cause has, as its etiologic fraction, the fraction of disease attributable to that sufficient cause (plus the fraction attributable to any other sufficient causes which contain the same component). Consider, for example, the causes schematically represented in figure 1. If Sufficient Cause I accounts for 50 per cent of a disease, Sufficient Cause II 30 per cent, and Sufficient Cause III 20 per cent, the etiologic fractions for each of the component causes are: A, 100 per cent; B, 80 per cent; C, 70 per cent; D, 50 per cent; E, 50 per cent; F, 50 per cent; G, 30 per cent; H, 30 per cent; I, 20 per cent; and J, 20 per cent. (The example would have to be modified slightly if there were individuals with more than one sufficient cause because for these people blocking one sufficient cause would not prevent disease.) This example illustrates that the sum of etiologic fractions of a set of factors is not limited above by unity, as is observed with alcohol and tobacco as etiologic agents for mouth cancer, each having an etiologic fraction greater than 50 per cent.

RISK

The notion of a risk as a continuous measure obscures the concept of risk as applied to an individual. For an individual, risk for disease properly defined takes on only two values: zero and unity. The application of some intermediate value for risk to an individual is only a means of estimating the individual's risk by the mean risk of many other presumably similar individuals. The actual risk for an individual is a matter of whether or not a sufficient cause has been or will be formed, whereas the mean risk for a group indicates the proportion of individuals for whom sufficient causes are formed. An individual's risk can be viewed as a probability statement about the likelihood of a sufficient cause for disease existing within the appropriate time frame.

STRENGTH OF A CAUSAL RISK FACTOR

The model proposed also illustrates how characterization of risk factors as "strong" or "weak" has no universal basis. A component cause which requires, to complete the sufficient cause, other components with low prevalence is thereby a "weak" (component) cause. The presence of such a component cause modifies the probability of the outcome only slightly, from zero to an average value just slightly greater than zero, reflecting the rarity of the complementary component causes. On the other hand, a component cause which requires, to complete the sufficient cause, other components which are nearly ubiquitous is a "strong" (component) cause. In epidemiologic terms, a weak cause confers only a small increment in disease risk, whereas a strong cause will increase disease risk substantially.

Thus the strength of a causal risk factor depends on the prevalence of the complementary component causes in the same sufficient cause. But this prevalence is often a matter of custom, circumstance or chance, and is not a scientifically generalizable characteristic. Consider the following simplified example (5): in a society where most people eat high phenylalanine diets, inheritance of the (rare) gene for PKU would appear to be a "strong" risk factor for phenylketonuric mental retardation, and phenylalanine in the diet would appear to be a weak risk factor. In another society, however, in which the gene for PKU is very common and few people eat high phenylalanine diets, inheritance of the gene would be a weak risk factor and phenylalanine in the diet would be a strong risk factor. Thus, the strength of a causal risk factor, as it might be measured by the "risk ratio" (relative risk) parameter, is dependent on the distribution in the population of the other causal factors in the same sufficient cause. The term *strength* of a causal risk factor retains some meaning as a description of the public health importance of a factor. However, the common epidemiologic parlance about strength of causal risk factors is devoid of meaning in the biologic description of disease etiology.

SYNERGY

Synergy, also termed effect modification or positive interaction, may be defined as the relationship between factors which exhibit a joint effect that exceeds the sum of the separate effects, with the effects measured on an appropriate scale (3,6). Synergy implies that two component causes are members of the same sufficient cause. Neither of two such causal components of a sufficient cause can have any effect (as part of that sufficient cause) without the presence of the other causal component. Two such causes, and, indeed, all the components of a given sufficient cause, are mutually synergistic. Thus, inheritance of the PKU gene and phenylalanine in the diet are synergistic in producing phenylketonuric mental retardation. If two causes are components of different sufficient causes for the same effect, and are not mutual members of any other sufficient cause for that effect, they will exhibit no synergy and are thus considered *independent* in the biologic (not statistical) sense. If two components of a sufficient cause have no effect outside that sufficient cause, they will exhibit complete synergy, in the sense that no increase in risk can occur from either factor unless both factors are present. It is commonly observed that causes seem to have less than complete synergy with other causes, because some increase in the probability for the effect is observed even when the causes occur in the absence of complementary, synergistic causes. This pattern results from such causes being members of more than one sufficient cause. Synergy results from component causes being mutual members of a sufficient cause, but the component causes each may also be members of other sufficient causes with different complements, thereby also having independent effects and making the overall interrelationship of two causes one of incomplete synergy. Thus, two factors may be mutual members of a sufficient cause, and each may separately be a member of another sufficient cause. Each factor in the absence of the other has an effect through one sufficient cause, but together they have an effect through three sufficient causes, displaying incomplete synergy. Necessary causes are at least partially synergistic with all other causes of the same effect, inasmuch as a necessary cause is a member of every sufficient cause.

Figure 1 suggests many synergistic relationships. For example, "D" and "E" are completely synergistic with each other and each is partially synergistic with "A", "B" and "C". Partial synergy exists between "B" and "C"—their effect is dependent on their joint presence in one sufficient cause, but each also has independent effects in another sufficient cause. The extent to which two factors are synergistic depends, like the strength of a causal risk factor, on the distribution of other factors in a particular population. Consider synergy between factors "B" and "F" in figure 1. This synergy results from both factors' presence in Sufficient Cause II, although "B" exerts a separate effect in Sufficient Cause I, and "F" in Sufficient Cause III. In a population where factor "H" were absent, "B" and "F" would exert their effects only through Sufficient Causes I and III, because the absence of "H" would eliminate any disease from Sufficient Cause II. Thus, "B" and "F" would be completely independent. In another population in which factor "C" were absent, all disease would result from Sufficient Cause II, and "B" and "F" would be fully synergistic.

An example of incomplete synergy would be the mixture of independent and interactive effects that alcohol consumption and smoking have on risk of mouth and pharynx cancer (7). Evidence suggests that either of these factors will increase cancer risk in the absence of the other, but the combined effect of both exceeds the sum of the individual effects. This would suggest at least three different causal complexes, one involving alcohol but not smoking, one involving smoking but not alcohol, and one involving both. (Some scientists have argued that alcohol in the absence of smoking has no effect, which leads to a model with two sufficient causes, one with smoking but not alcohol, and another with both smoking and alcohol.)

DISCUSSION

The conceptual scheme in figure 1 could be modified to permit greater complexity. Antagonistic causes might be included as a part of causal chains which lead to an element being included in a sufficient cause; the joint action of the components of a sufficient cause could be considered an effect with its own constellations of sufficient causes. Alternatively, the different "pies" in figure 1 might be constructed as a sequence of causal events, with branching pathways representing those segments of pies which differ, necessary causes being common to all pathways, etc. The possibilities for adapting this framework to virtually any complicated causal relationship reinforce its utility as an intuitive base for causal thinking.

The model also provides a conceptual framework for the understanding of *latent period*, the time interval between the action of a (component) cause and the manifestation of disease. When a component cause "acts" or occurs, the other components needed to complete a sufficient cause may not be on hand. If the component cause of interest has a long-lasting "effect", as time passes the other complementary components may add their "effects" and gradually complete the sufficient cause. At the point in time at which the sufficient cause is completed, the disease process is set in motion, though usually not yet manifest. The latent period is the interval during which a sufficient cause accumulates plus the time it takes for disease to become manifest. Early recognition could theoretically reduce the latent period to coincide with the interval during which the sufficient cause accumulates.

For some diseases, such as rabies, virtually the entire period from internalizing the viral agent to the occurrence of symptoms represents time during which the disease becomes manifest, because "internalizing" the viral agent is effectively a sufficient cause (a qualification would be that interventive treatment during the "incubation" period might prevent clinical manifestation). On the other hand, the larger part of the 10–20-year latent period for the development of vaginal cancer after *in utero*

592   KENNETH J. ROTHMAN

exposure to diethylstilbesterol probably represents accumulation of a sufficient cause (which might ordinarily be completed at menarche or during adolescence) with only a few years for the disease to become manifest after the sufficient cause is complete. The term *incubation period* has often been applied to the period between the accumulation of a sufficient cause and the time at which disease becomes manifest. Because reversal of disease may be possible during the preclinical development, as in the example of rabies treatment, or catalysts may act to shorten the incubation period of diseases which might otherwise fester in a preclinical state interminably (growth enhancers for neoplasms are an example), it might be better to view the latent period as solely the accumulation of a sufficient cause, components of which might include developmental catalysts and/or the lack of interventive treatment.

Chronic exposures make it more difficult to quantify, and, indeed, to conceptualize latent period; different doses of an exposure accumulated over time may give rise to different risks. Such situations may be viewed as reflecting a set of different sufficient causes, each with a different dose of the exposure as a component cause. Small doses would presumably require a more complex set of complementary component causes to complete the sufficient cause than large doses. This extension of the causal model accommodates the description of dose-response relationships, and provides a basis for the common finding that for many carcinogens the dose is related directly to risk and inversely to latent period.

This presentation does not treat the subtle issues which arise in arriving at a workable definition of disease. Such issues obviously pertain to a full consideration of causes, inasmuch as disease definition may be based on experiential criteria (8), but these considerations go beyond the scope of this paper.

It might be argued that the scheme presented here is superficial because the occurrence of disease in any individual involves a collection of component causes which constitute a sufficient cause that is unique, by its complexity. Individually unique sufficient causes, however, would detract equally from all generalized causal models. Furthermore, despite individual distinctions it seems likely that there would be broad similarities in the components of sufficient causes for different individuals.

REFERENCES

1. Elandt-Johnson RC: Definition of rates: Some remarks on their use and misuse. Am J Epidemiol 102:267–271, 1975
2. Miettinen OS: Confounding and effect modification. Am J Epidemiol 100:350–353, 1974
3. Rothman KJ: Synergy and antagonism in cause-effect relationships. Am J Epidemiol 99:385–388, 1974
4. Miettinen OS: Proportion of disease caused or prevented by a given exposure, trait, or intervention. Am J Epidemiol 99:325–332, 1974
5. MacMahon B: Gene-environment interaction in human disease. J Psychiat Res 6 (supp 1):393–402, 1968
6. Rothman KJ: Estimation of synergy and antagonism. Am J Epidemiol 103:506–511, 1976
7. Rothman KJ, Keller AZ: The effect of joint exposure to alcohol and tobacco on risk of cancer of the mouth and pharynx. J. Chronic Dis 25:711–716, 1972
8. MacMahon B, Pugh TF. Epidemiology. Principles and Methods. Boston, Little, Brown and Company, 1970

I–8.

A Series of Exchanges on Popperian Philosophy in Epidemiology:

Carol Buck: Popper's Philosophy for Epidemiologists.
International Journal of Epidemiology 1975; 4:159–168.

With Replies by: A. Michael Davies (Int J Epidemiol 1975; 4:169–171),
Alwyn Smith (Int J Epidemiol 1975; 4:171–172),
Andrew Creese (Int J Epidemiol 1975; 4:352–353),
Richard Peto (Int J Epidemiol 1976; 5:97), and
Carol Buck (Int J Epidemiol 1976; 5:97–98).

M. Jacobsen: Against Popperized Epidemiology.
International Journal of Epidemiology 1976; 5:9–11.

I had been exposed to the writings of Karl Popper and Thomas Kuhn as an undergraduate, but their views came to life for me with their appearance in the epidemiologic literature in the mid-1970's. The debate over the value and meaning of Popper's philosophy for epidemiology continues (see, e.g., Am J Epidemiol 1986; 123:199, 965, and 1119), but the following exchange from the *International Journal of Epidemiology* inspired a broader search for methodologic insights from the philosophy of science, in addition to fueling the debate over whether epidemiology should regard itself as a branch of science or public health. Of course, the exchange settled nothing and so I will refrain from commenting on it, but I recommend the following readings to those intrigued by the philosophical issues:

Brown HI. *Perception, Theory, and Commitment.* Chicago: Precedent Publishing Inc., 1977.
Kuhn TS. *The Structure of Scientific Revolutions.* Second edition. Chicago: University of Chicago Press, 1970.
Lakatos I, Musgrave A, eds. *Criticism and the Growth of Knowledge.* New York: Cambridge University Press, 1970.
Miller D, ed. *Popper Selections.* Princeton: Princeton University Press, 1985.
Popper KR. *The Logic of Scientific Discovery.* New York: Harper and Row, 1968.

International Journal of Epidemiology
© Oxford University Press 1975

Vol. 4, No. 3
Printed in Great Britain

Popper's Philosophy for Epidemiologists

CAROL BUCK[1]

Buck, C. (Dept. Epidemiology and Preventive Medicine, University of Western Ontario, London 72, Canada). Popper's philosophy for epidemiologists. *Int. J. Epid.* 1975, **4**: 159–168.
This paper discusses the application of Popper's philosophy to epidemiological research, examining in particular the problems of replication without risk of refutation, of mistaking statistical sophistication for deductive inference, and of dealing with causality at a general level. An example is given of a Popperian approach to the test of a causal hypothesis concerning cancer of the cervix.

INTRODUCTION

Bryan Magee (1) opens his book on Popper with the remark that *Karl Popper is not, as yet anyway, a household name among the educated.* Nor is his a household name among scientists, few of whom are interested in the philosophy of scientific inquiry. Although many have been given an introduction to the logical foundations of science during their training, only a minority renew the acquaintance. This is unfortunate, particularly at present when there are signs of an impending withdrawal of the *carte blanche* that for so long has been offered to science. We hear protests against the lavish financial support given to investigators among whom only a few are capable of creative work. The suggestion has been made more than once that mediocre scientists no longer be given even modest research funds and that instead they be put to work in a supporting capacity with demonstrably creative investigators. I think it possible that among the apparently mediocre there is a significant number who could be creative were they aware of Popper's philosophy of science. Productive habits of thought might be acquired if thought were given more emphasis and action less.

Platt (2) says that one of the outstanding differences between productive and unproductive branches of science is the use of strong inference in the former. By this he means the orderly progression from hypothesis to prediction and then to observation as a way of discarding and revising hypotheses. Although Platt mentions Popper only in passing, it is Popper's philosophy that he prescribes. *How many of us write down our alternatives and crucial experiments every day, focusing*

---

[1] Professor of Epidemiology and Preventive Medicine, University of Western Ontario, London 72, Canada.

on the exclusion *of a hypothesis? . . . We become 'method-oriented' rather than 'problem-oriented'. We say we prefer to 'feel our way' toward generalizations. We fail to teach our students to sharpen up their inductive inferences. And we do not realize the added power that the regular and explicit use of alternative hypotheses and sharp exclusions could give us at every step of our research. The difference between the average scientist's informal methods and the methods of the strong inference users is somewhat like the difference between a gasoline engine that fires occasionally and one that fires in steady sequence. If our motor engines were as erratic as our deliberate intellectual efforts, most of us would not get home for supper* (2).

Slater (3) has summarized Popper's philosophy for the benefit of investigators in psychiatry, a field in which the line between art and science is particularly difficult to draw. The difference between the failings of psychiatry on the one hand and those of the biological medical sciences on the other is interesting. Bad science in psychiatry usually arises from the creation of a global hypothesis which is poetically elaborated upon by its creator and his followers without any appeal to facts that would be capable of refuting it. Bad science in medical biology usually arises from an investigator behaving as a naturalist and applying technically ingenious methods to the collection of observations that test no hypothesis. For both such tendencies Popper supplies a powerful remedy.

Since my purpose is to discuss the application of Popper's philosophy to epidemiology, I shall make no further gratuitous comments about the failing of other branches of medical science. What shortcomings do we have that attention to Popper might correct?

Epidemiologists are exceptionally concerned about their method of approach. In few other medical sciences is so much attention devoted to the philosophical, as opposed to the purely technical, aspect of method. The reason for this is that in epidemiology the experiment plays a relatively minor role. It is usually necessary to create a quasi-experiment out of naturally occurring phenomena. The dangers inherent in a quasi-experiment have made epidemiologists especially attentive to the logical foundations of their work. But their concern with logical rigour is narrow in a Popperian sense and could be raised to a more creative level if Popper's views were better known. Had I encountered Popper's writings earlier, I would have done many things differently.

A SUMMARY OF POPPER'S PHILOSOPHY*

The traditional view of science has been that induction, the formation of a hypothesis based upon observation, is the mainstay of the scientific process. This has always presented a logical difficulty because a hypothesis so derived is forever vulnerable to denial by the first observation that proves an exception. If by induction we believe that all swans are white, our belief can be overthrown by one appearance of a black swan. Popper has rejected the traditional view and regards induction as a dispensable concept. He believes that all observations are made to test some hypothesis already in mind, the derivation of the hypothesis being a work of the imagination. One uses deductive reasoning to make predictions from the hypothesis and thus to state what it prohibits. Scientific discovery in Popper's view is based solely upon a hypothetico-deductive process and advances by disproof rather than proof.

Sherlock Holmes said that *when you have eliminated the impossible whatever remains, however improbable, must be the truth*. This aphorism nearly summarizes Popper's philosophy, except that 'must' in the last phrase should be altered to 'may'.

Given that knowledge is advanced only by testing hypotheses and discarding those that fail, the value of a hypothesis depends upon the degree to which testable and thus refutable predictions can

be made from it. A useful hypothesis, therefore, has two important characteristics:

(i) The phenomena that it predicts are open to observation. In fact, if a hypothesis lacks this characteristic it lies outside the boundary of science.

(ii) It is rich in empirical content and so identifies many phenomena that would be incompatible with it.

If a new hypothesis is advanced in competition with one currently held, we should prefer the new hypothesis if at least one of the following criteria is satisfied:

(i) It makes more precise predictions;
(ii) It explains more of the previous observations;
(iii) It explains the previous observations in more detail;
(iv) It has passed tests which the older hypothesis has failed;
(v) It has suggested new tests (i.e. made new predictions) not suggested by the older hypothesis;
(vi) It has unified or connected phenomena not previously considered to be related.

The first, fourth and fifth criteria are most specifically Popperian. The second, third and sixth are familiar as components of the general tenet of scientific parsimony. All are superior to the vague advice often given to scientists that the 'simplest' theory should be preferred.

These criteria emphasize the need to advance beyond the purely *ad hoc* hypothesis that explains a phenomenon equally well but no better than an older hypothesis. For as Popper says, it is always possible to produce a theory to fit any set of observations. We advance only when we suggest refutable consequences of the theory. As long as this requirement is met, there is nothing wrong in forming an *a posteriori* hypothesis because a prior hypothesis was completely contradicted by the observations made to test it. In an epidemiological study of the influence of season of conception upon the IQ of the offspring, Knobloch and Pasamanick (4) observed a relationship almost exactly the opposite of the one that their theory predicted. They were criticized (5) for immediately switching hypotheses in order to explain what had been observed. The criticism is to some extent justified, but only because they put forward few suggestions for refuting their new hypothesis.

---

* The reader who wishes to go beyond this summary can turn to any one of three books by Karl Popper: 1. *The Logic of Scientific Discovery*, 2nd ed., Harper & Rowe, New York, 1968; 2. *Conjectures and Refutations*, 4th ed., Routledge & Kegan Paul, London, 1972; 3. *Objective Knowledge: An Evolutionary Approach*, Oxford University Press, London, 1972.

To those who find Popper's approach congenial, it may seem that such a view of science is self-evident and that Popper can hardly be credited with having created a new philosophy of science. Medawar in *The Art of the Soluble* (6) raised this question and pointed out that William Whewell of Trinity College, Cambridge, had expressed as early as 1840 a view very similar to Popper's when he stated that the failure to refute a hypothesis *after trying to do so* was much more significant than the mere absence of known facts that were incompatible with it. Similarly, Lord Acton (7) in 1895 stressed the importance of considering objections to a theory: *Remember Darwin taking note of only those passages that raised difficulties in his way; the French philosopher complaining that his work stood still because he found no more contradicting facts; Baer who thinks error treated thoroughly, nearly as remunerative as truth, by the discovery of new objections; for as Sir Robert Ball warns us, it is by considering objections that we often learn.* Coming closer to our own field, we have the following statement from Karl Pearson (8): *The assumption which lies at the bottom of most popular fallacious inference might pass without reference for it is obviously absurd, were it not, alas! so widely current. The assumption is simply this: that the strongest argument in favour of the truth of a statement is the absence or impossibility of a demonstration of its falsehood.* Thus Popper has distinguished forebears. It is he, however, who has described the hypothetico-deductive method in fullest detail and has given the most rigorous logical reasons for adopting it.

Just at a time when Popper's philosophy has been attracting more general attention, there appeared in the popular scientific literature the work of Edward de Bono (9). His essays on creative thinking provide a useful companion to the work of Popper. To search for all the refutable consequences of a hypothesis demands highly imaginative thinking. Imagination is needed to arrive at the hypothesis in the first place, let alone to suggest rigorous tests for it. Although imaginative thinking is commonly regarded as an inborn ability which cannot be taught, de Bono suggests many techniques for enhancing whatever abilities a person has received from nature. His Popperian approach is well illustrated by the following quotation from *The Use of Lateral Thinking*:

Every decision is made with some degree of uncertainty. Confidence in a decision does not depend on the lack of any alternative, for that might only indicate lack of imagination, but on the ability to see many alternatives all of which can be rejected. In the making of any decision it can be useful to use one's own or someone else's lateral thinking to generate alternative views so that rejection of these can strengthen the decision. A free-thinking devil's advocate, instead of casting doubts on a good decision, can only succeed in strengthening it.

De Bono also offers this appealing example of the untestable *ad hoc* hypothesis: *Sects which assemble on mountain tops on predicted days of doom to await the end of the world do not come down on the morrow shaken in their ideas, but with a renewed faith in the mercifulness of the Almighty.*

Popper's tenets are more compelling to the intellect than to the emotions. The creator of a hypothesis is inclined to have a personal attachment to his creature and is not intuitively disposed to seek eagerly for a means of refuting it. Platt has suggested that it is easier to follow Popper's criterion of falsifiability if one makes multiple hypotheses to explain a phenomenon. Indeed, as Lakatos emphasizes (10), the importance of Popper's philosophy lies in its use of refutability to choose which among competing hypotheses should be pursued rather than to reject hastily any single theory. De Bono makes the further point that the exercise of developing multiple hypotheses improves one's capacity for imaginative thought and thus increases the likelihood of arriving at a highly innovative hypothesis.

The importance of breaking the habit of clinging to and endlessly buttressing a single hypothesis is richly illustrated by research on cigarette smoking. Here hypotheses are embraced with such fervour that the thought of refutability becomes heresy. Yerushalmy (11) deserved great credit for his ingenious attempt to test the causal significance of smoking in low birthweight by comparing babies born before and after their mother took up the smoking habit. Yet his readers have paid far less attention to the ingenuity of his approach than to the confounding effect of maternal age which made his results inconclusive. I think that their attitude can be explained by the exasperation created among epidemiologists by ignorant and sometimes corrupt defenders of smoking. In such an emotional climate, it is very easy to abandon Popper's cardinal precept that refutation is heuristically more powerful than confirmation.

THE APPLICATION OF POPPER'S PHILOSOPHY TO EPIDEMIOLOGY

In Popper's terms, the formation of some hypotheses, however preliminary, precedes the collection of data on the distribution of a disease. The data must be capable of refuting the hypothesis. By judicious oscillation between the making of hypotheses and the gathering of data, epidemiologists should be able to discard many hypotheses without recourse to experiment. The experiment, always a most difficult undertaking in epidemiology, is reserved for testing the hypothesis that has survived ingenious deductive efforts to falsify it in observational studies.

Modern epidemiology, concerned with all kinds of illness and not just with communicable disease, is a relatively new branch of medical science. Consequently its aims are not always well understood. How frequently we hear the request to *give us the epidemiology of disease X*, by which is meant an account of the time trend of X and the way in which its frequency is related to age, sex, geographical area, occupation and other demographic variables. I fear that too often this is all that is expected of epidemiology. A commonly held view is that the epidemiologist gathers data from which other scientists will build hypotheses. This view excludes epidemiologists from the exciting process of scientific deduction, and puts them into the business of induction which Popper so convincingly dismisses as irrelevant.

Some epidemiologists appear content with this arrangement. Some get around it by working collaboratively with other scientists so that they may participate in the deductive process. Some, especially those who are medically qualified, go directly to the literature of another branch of medicine in order to construct their own hypotheses. A recent example of the last can be found in the work of Anderson (12). He reached his hypothesis about the role of dietary antioxidants in myocardial infarction by studying the literature on muscular dystrophy, realizing that the latter might be analogous to the myocardial response to ischaemia.

The epidemiologists who are content to serve as preliminary data-gatherers should not be criticized, as long as they are there by choice and not by a mistakenly diffident view of the role of epidemiology in medical science. The two avenues of escape open to an epidemiologist who is not content with data-gathering are probably equally acceptable. What matters is that epidemiologists be fully aware of the part that they could play in the scientific process.

Three features of epidemiological research are particularly worthy of examination from Popper's point of view.

1. *The problem of replication without risk of refutation*

The collection of data is an indispensable part of the epidemiological process, but it can become a wasteful activity if it is not inspired by a deductive aim.

If an epidemiological study in one country has shown that a disease is related to a particular set of variables, why should another epidemiologist repeat the study in his own country? There are only two legitimate reasons. The first has to do with the need to confirm observations because the play of chance can create spurious associations. The role of chance can never be eliminated, but can be given a measure of probability from tests of statistical significance with whose logic epidemiologists are better acquainted than most medical scientists. A large probability that chance explains an association may derive from a paucity of observations. Here, then, is one justification for replication of an epidemiological study. When this is the purpose, the replication should be as exact a reproduction as is possible of the original study. Wilson (13) has criticized epidemiologists for failing either to undertake or to publish when it is called for.

The second reason for replication is deductively much more powerful in Popper's sense. Suppose one hypothesizes that an endogenous degenerative process plays a major causative role in a disease. A positive association of the disease with age would support the hypothesis. But the identification of a population in which age had no relationship to the disease would suggest the alternative hypothesis that it is caused by prolonged exposure to an exogenous factor, present in some populations and absent in others. The greater one's age, the longer would be one's exposure to the factor if it were present. Repetition of a study that showed age-dependency thus should be made in a population as different as possible from the original one. Replication then becomes an attempt at refutation. If the study is repeated in a population little different from that in which the association with age was first observed, no serious attempt is being made to refute a hypothesis. After many confirmations of the positive relationship between hypertension and age, it was rather belatedly realized (14) that in some populations the relationship is absent. With an earlier search for such exceptions and a vigorous pursuit of the alternative hypothesis that they suggest, our knowledge of the causes of hypertension might now be further ahead.

Thus an epidemiologist must consider carefully his reason for repeating the work of others. Is the reason a statistical one, to decrease the role of chance in an association, or is it a deductive one, to identify circumstances under which the association does not exist? Sometimes the latter has already been accomplished but has gone unheeded. Consider for example, the well-known positive relationship between latitude and multiple sclerosis, which has been variously interpreted as reflecting the importance of sunshine, diet or race. Japan's low rate was regarded as a tolerable inconsistency until Poskanzer and his colleagues (15) seized upon this as a basis for a new hypothesis, namely that poliomyelitis in the adult is a precursor of multiple sclerosis. The new hypothesis would explain Japan's aberrantly low frequency of multiple sclerosis in terms of its previously 'tropical' pattern of poliomyelitis (widespread infection in childhood and subsequent immunity in adults).

The epidemiological investigation of coronary artery disease offers another example. Many studies have been made, in very similar populations, of the physiological and psychological correlates of heart disease. The number of nearly identical investigations now exceeds the statistical requirement for replication of their common findings. Many of them have been undertaken without any intent to test predictions based upon competing hypotheses. Yet their discordant findings with respect to the association between coronary artery disease and socio-economic status could have led much earlier to the formation of new hypotheses, such as the interesting one that it is status incongruity rather than socio-economic level that plays a causal role in coronary disease (16).

The wastefulness of epidemiological research that has no deductive impetus has been emphasized in a recent paper by Neri, Hewitt and Schreiber (17), in which they discuss the relation between water hardness and mortality. The title itself is interesting, *Can Epidemiology Elucidate the Water Story?* They refer to four classes of hypotheses concerning the apparently protective effect of hard water. The first category deals with a purely indirect role of hard water arising from its association with other factors related to mortality. The second deals with bulk protective ingredients in hard water, the third with trace protective elements and the fourth with harmful factors in soft water. They say that it is inconceivable that one research design would provide a basis for discriminating among all four categories and that epidemiologists should forsake their hopes of bringing off a scientific *coup* and be content to ensure that their projected studies have at least some discriminatory power among the four kinds of hypotheses. After reviewing fifty studies of water hardness in relation to mortality, they conclude that half had no discriminatory power at all and that the rest were mainly concerned with discriminating between a general and a cardio-specific effect of hard water. They finish with the remark that *epidemiological studies will have something to contribute if conducted . . . with due regard for specifying and testing explicit hypotheses.*

Although Popper's philosophy requires that a new hypothesis should explain previous observations, it demands more than this. If an epidemiologist tests his hypothesis against existing observations and finds it compatible with all of them, he cannot stop there without falling into the trap of *ad hoc* reasoning. Yet the exercise of reviewing a hypothesis in the light of previous observations is useful because it provides an inexpensive preliminary exposure to refutation. The proper use of this exercise is illustrated by Matthews and Glasse (18). After testing against all the facts their hypothesis that the tropical disease Kuru is infectious rather than genetic in origin, they made a prediction about the future incidence of Kuru in New Guinea after cannibalism has ceased. On the fulfilment of this prediction their hypothesis now rests.

Epidemiologists are sometimes asked why John Snow invariably receives the greatest prominence in any historical account of their subject. The simple reason is that he was successful in establishing a causal mechanism for an important disease and that he accomplished this by methods that we now call epidemiological. What needs more emphasis in our praise of Snow is the consistently deductive nature of his approach. When he gathered new data, it was always for the purpose of testing a highly specific prediction of his hypothesis. The incident of the Broad Street pump in Soho has become famous as one of the first experiments in epidemiology (19). Snow's recommendation that the pump be closed may not have been viewed by him as an experiment so much as a mandatory action. Having shown that people living beyond the area of the pump who had used its water were attacked, while residents of the area who did not drink from it were spared, what other action could have been recommended? In my view, Snow should be revered more for his analytical epidemiology than for his famous experiment.

2. *The problem of mistaking statistical sophistication for strong inference*

Because epidemiologists are sophisticated in analytical methods, it is very easy for them to believe that they are doing better than most medical scientists in following Popper's principle of falsifiability. I refer here to the epidemiological craft of dealing with confounding and intervening variables, which has been well expounded in Susser's book, *Causal Thinking in the Health Sciences* (20). However, one must realize that there is a vital difference between the usual exercise of this craft and Popper's principle of testing a hypothesis by searching for its refutable predictions.

The separation of confounding variables is an important technique for determining whether we have a new hypothesis or whether we are merely restating a previously established relationship. It can also be useful for analysing observations that have been made to test the predicted consequences of a new hypothesis. But since it is only a technique it should be the servant not the master of our imagination. This point needs to be put forcefully to students of epidemiology who can easily be led by their teachers to believe that the analytical methods of epidemiology are an end in themselves.

An excessive recourse to statistical devices for tidying up epidemiological data may cause us to miss the exception that in Popper's sense tests the rule. Miettinen (21) has recently shown how by standardizing and summarizing stratified data we can obscure important modifiers of cause and effect relationships.

Adherence to Popper's principle of starting with a hypothesis will protect the epidemiologist from the pitfalls of multivariate analysis. In the absence of a specific hypothesis it is all too easy to emerge from such an analysis with a set of near-zero regression coefficients. This gives the false impression that something has been refuted when in fact all that has been accomplished is the statistical formulation of a tautology. If, however, a multivariate procedure is undertaken to test a carefully formulated hypothesis, we are more likely to put into the equation variables that are conceptually distinct from one another and therefore amenable to statistical separation.

The epidemiologist's preoccupation with methodological niceties may sometimes cause the premature rejection of a hypothesis that should be pursued. Fliess (22), with a viewpoint different from mine, mentions Raymond Pearl's suggestion in 1929 that the protein of the tubercle bacillus might be curative of cancer. Pearl's suggestion arose from his observation that cancer and tuberculosis were rarely associated. Because his observation was based on autopsy data it was dismissed, perhaps too hastily, as an example of Berkson's fallacy. Yet now, nearly 50 years later, BCG is being tested as a treatment for cancer. The irony of this cannot escape even the most methodologically compulsive epidemiologist.

3. *The problem of dealing with causality at the general level*

In the epidemiological study of chronic disease, work usually begins at such a broad level of causality that the predictions of a hypothesis have to be couched in vague terms. Consequently the observations capable of refuting the predictions may be difficult to specify. Unless we realize this, we are in danger of applying the principle of falsification at the naive level against which Lakatos (10) warns the recent convert to Popper. If the predictions of a theory fail to be upheld by observations that are themselves inappropriate, no useful refutation has been accomplished. Let us again take multiple sclerosis as an example, this time with the measles virus as a supposed causal factor. Few of us would think it appropriate to regard the absence of measles antibodies in some patients as a phenomenon prohibited by the hypothesis and therefore as a test of its validity. More likely an epidemiologist would postulate that other factors were also capable of inducing multiple sclerosis. A more appropriate test would then be based on the prediction that epidemics of measles would be followed after some defined interval by an increase in the frequency of multiple sclerosis. But this prediction could lead to difficulty if several common viruses were causally involved. A rise in multiple sclerosis due to measles might be obscured by concomitant decreases in the incidence of the other viral infections. With some knowledge of immunology, the epidemiologist might hypothesize that the antigenic properties of a set of viruses, to which measles belongs, provoke an aberrant immune response that may result in multiple sclerosis. The prediction could then be restated in terms that would permit a more meaningful refutation.

In their textbook of epidemiology, MacMahon and Pugh (23) say that a causal hypothesis based upon epidemiological evidence is strengthened if it invokes some known, or at least possible, physiological mechanism. Although their book contains many Popperian ideas, they would be even more in tune with Popper if they said that a physiological mechanism is useful in suggesting a means of refuting the hypothesis.

Another example of the difficult early stages of epidemiological research can be drawn from psychiatry. Much work has gone into the search for environmental causes of mental illness, with the putative causes expressed in only the most general terms. If a prediction is made at this level in order to test a hypothesis, its refutation may have little value. Take for example the remarkable variability in the results of inquiries into the relationship between loss of a parent in childhood and subsequent mental illness. Such variability could easily lead to spurious refutation of a hypothesis that depended upon finding the relationship. Birtchnell (24) explains the variability by noting that there are many possible consequences of bereavement and that these undoubtedly vary according to other features of the bereaved child's situation. This and other examples of global variables lead him to a conclusion that is essentially a hopeless one for epidemiology, but not a surprising one in view of the title of his paper: *Is There a Scientifically Acceptable Alternative to the Epidemiological Study of Familial Factors in Mental Illness?* I do not share his view that epidemiologists must be confined to the study of global variables. If they appreciate the need, surely they can refine a global variable into its deductively more powerful components.

Cassel (25) offers an excellent illustration of the need to make a hypothesis as rich as possible, even if its components are rather global in nature. He cites a study in which it was predicted that life-stress would increase the risk of complications among pregnant women who lacked the social support necessary to deal with stress. The study confirmed the prediction. But had either of two simpler hypotheses been formed their predictions would have been refuted, because neither life-stress nor social support was related to complications of pregnancy when considered alone.

The foregoing examples take me back to a point touched upon earlier. Can the epidemiologist, unless he specializes in a particular disease, construct hypotheses for which productive refutation is possible? It is easier to specialize than repeatedly to find expert collaborators as one moves from disease to disease. The latter may be preferable, however, from the standpoint of creativity.

Returning to de Bono (9), we hear from him convincing arguments for not specializing. He believes that a creative hypothesis is more likely to occur to a person not so saturated by conventional ways of regarding a phenomenon that he is unable to look at it upside down and backwards.

There is nevertheless an advantage to be gained from the very general level of causality at which epidemiologists frequently operate. At this level it may be possible to apply another of Popper's criteria, namely that a strong theory unifies or connects hitherto unrelated problems. Cassel (25) took this viewpoint when he suggested that epidemiologists might be more productive if they worked sometimes from cause to disease rather than in the more usual reverse direction. He suggested, for example, that the rapid urbanization and industrialization of a rural population might produce stress that enhanced susceptibility to many diseases. I think this approach has been discouraged by the distaste of epidemiologists for a putative causal factor that 'causes too much'. In an attempt to generalize from Koch's postulates for establishing causality in microbial disease, it has been said that one should be wary of a factor that appears to play a part in many diseases. If this advice had been taken seriously at the time when the various symptoms of lead poisoning were regarded as separate diseases, an appreciation of the toxic nature of lead would have been greatly delayed. As Susser (20) suggests, we would be more faithful to Koch's real meaning if we predicted the specific cause-effect relationships embodied in a 'super-cause'.

AN EXERCISE IN THE POPPERIAN APPROACH TO EPIDEMIOLOGY

Let us look at the history of the epidemiological investigation of cancer of the uterine cervix. In 1948, Kennaway (26) published his painstaking compilation and imaginative interpretation of data concerning cancer of the uterus. He concluded with the following statement: *The data collected in this paper suggest the existence of two factors which may increase the incidence of cancer of the uterus, namely:*

(1) *A factor which is opposed by the Jewish practice of abstention from intercourse during most of the first half of the ovulatory cycle, and*

(2) *A factor intensified in both married and single women by descent in the economic scale.*

As the investigation of cancer of the cervix continued, it became clear that the age of beginning sexual intercourse was another factor, with the risk of cervical cancer elevated among women who began intercourse under the age of 17.

In 1968, 20 years after Kennaway's paper, Rawls (27) advanced evidence in favour of the hypothesis that a venerally transmitted virus (Herpes type 2) is the carcinogenic agent.

The infectious hypothesis is compatible with the social class gradient of cancer of the cervix. It is also compatible with the fact that the disease is more strongly associated with the number of sexual partners than with the frequency of sexual intercourse, a point made by Terris (28) when he discussed infectious versus chemical carcinogenesis as a cause of cervical cancer.

The infectious hypothesis has been made to embrace the association with age at first intercourse by appending to it one of the following:

(a) the adolescent cervix is more susceptible to viral infection;
(b) the adolescent cervix is more susceptible to viral carcinogenesis;
(c) first coitus under age 17 is associated with promiscuity and therefore with high exposure to infection.

The last fits poorly with Terris' finding that women with multiple sexual partners were at greater risk of cervical cancer only if they married after the age of 17.

By what explanation can the infectious hypothesis be reconciled with the remarkable sparing of Jews? The protection against infection afforded by circumcision is an unlikely explanation because the importance of circumcision in cancer of the cervix is negligible among non-Jewish women. Martin (29) has suggested that the endogamy practised by Jews creates a barrier to the entrance of an infectious agent into Jewish populations. Or, an explanation based upon racial immunity to infection might be invoked. The last explanation would be difficult to accept in the face of the equally low frequency of cervical cancer among Ashkenazi and Sephardic Jews in Israel (30). These two groups of Jews have been geographically separated for a long period of time, they differ in certain anthropometric indices, and they have a markedly different incidence of a genetic disorder, Tay-Sachs disease (31).

As an exercise in Popperian epidemiology, I shall restate the infectious hypothesis so that it unites the observations about age at first intercourse and abstention from intercourse by orthodox Jews during much of the pre-ovulatory phase of the menstrual cycle. The revised hypothesis is this:

susceptibility of the cervical epithelium to viral carcinogenesis is greatest in the first few years after menarche and in the pre-ovulatory phase of the menstrual cycle, because at both times the cervix lacks the protective effect of progesterone. At the menarche, anovulatory cycles are common and are only gradually replaced in the ensuing 2–3 years by ovulatory cycles in which progesterone counteracts oestrogen-induced changes in the cervical epithelium.

The next step in the exercise is to make as many testable predictions as possible from the re-stated hypothesis. I have made the following eight predictions:

1. Cancer of the cervix among Jewish women should occur mainly among those who do not observe the orthodox sexual ritual.

Stewart *et al.* found that among Jewish women, fewer cases than controls abstained from intercourse during the first week after the menses (30). The proportion stating that they observed the full sexual ritual (Laws of Niddah) was not, however, greater in the controls. In Israel, Pridan and Lilienfeld found no difference between cases and controls in the woman's own assessment of her orthodoxy in religion (32).

2. The beginning of sexual relations at an early age should be a more important risk factor in cervical cancer among orthodox Jewish women than among all other women, because the sexual ritual of the former affords protection once ovulatory cycles have been established.

This prediction receives some support from Stewart *et al.*, whose data show a much greater difference between cases and controls in median age at first intercourse among Israeli Jewish women than among New York Jewish or non-Jewish women (30). On the other hand, Pridan and Lilienfeld found only a small difference between their Israeli cases and controls in the proportion beginning intercourse under the age of 20 (32).

3. Among orthodox Jewish women who did not begin sexual activity at an early age, there should be no social class gradient in the incidence of cervical cancer. After ovulation has been established, the protection afforded by the Jewish sexual ritual would override any differences in hygiene associated with social class.

Pridan and Lilienfeld (32) found little evidence of a social class trend in their case-control study of

Jewish women, although they did not examine the relationship according to age at first intercourse.

4. Among orthodox Jewish women, the number of marital partners should not be an important risk factor in cervical cancer, because the Jewish sexual ritual would make exposure to infection irrelevant.

In Pridan and Lilienfeld's study, the number of marital partners was not important, except among Jewish women emigrating to Israel after 1955 (32). If the more recent immigrants were less orthodox, this observation would be consistent with the prediction. But if exposure to infection can be increased by the sexual activity of either marital partner, the prediction is not supported by their observation that husbands of cases had more sexual partners than husbands of controls.

Nor is this prediction fully supported by data from the New York-Israel study showing number of marital partners according to age at first marriage (30). Among women marrying at age 20 or later, the difference between cases and controls in the number of marital partners was smaller among Jewish women in Israel than among Jewish women in New York. However, the difference was equally small among non-Jewish women in New York.

5. In a case-control study of women who began coitus at an early age, the age at menarche should be later among the cases in order for a higher proportion of their sexual activity to have occurred during the phase of anovulatory cycles.

Stewart *et al.* (30) provide some data to test this prediction. The proportion of women beginning intercourse under the age of 20 is given according to age at menarche. The prediction is not borne out, because the difference between cases and controls in age at first intercourse was not at a maximum among women with late menarche.

6. The beginning of sexual relations before the age of 17 should be less strongly related to cervical cancer among women who bore children prior to that age, because their average age of establishing ovulatory cycles will have been earlier. I have found no data for testing this prediction.

7. A history of repeated spontaneous abortion should be associated with cervical cancer, because susceptibility to abortion is to some extent related to low levels of progesterone. The validity of this prediction rests on the assumption that the pro-

gesterone level in pregnancy is correlated with that during the normal menstrual cycle.

Rotkin (33) provides some evidence against the prediction. He found no difference between cases and controls in the overall frequency of abortion. But if habitual aborters are only a small proportion of all women with at least one spontaneous abortion, his observation does not entirely refute this prediction.

8. The incidence of cervical cancer in various Jewish populations should be highly correlated with their degree of orthodoxy.

I have put this prediction last because unless one makes bizarre assumptions about the extent of Jewish orthodoxy in the United States, it is resoundingly refuted by the equal incidence of cervical cancer among Jewish women in Israel and New York (30). Had this prediction been considered first, there would have been little point in continuing the exercise.

Although the exercise has supplied no clue to the epidemiological puzzle of cancer of the cervix, I hope that it has illustrated Popper's approach to the construction and demolition of a hypothesis.

ACKNOWLEDGEMENTS

I would like to thank Dr. Kathleen Stavraky and Professor Carl Robinow for their helpful comments on the first draft of this paper.

REFERENCES

(1) Magee, B.: *Popper*. London: Fontana/Collins, 1973.
(2) Platt, J. R.: Strong inference. *Science* **146**: 347, 1964.
(3) Slater, E.: The psychiatrist in search of a science. *Brit. J. Psychiatry* **122**: 625, 1973.
(4) Knobloch, H. and Pasamanick, B.: Seasonal variation in the births of the mentally deficient. *Amer. J. Pub. Health* **48**: 1201, 1958.
(5) Sterling, T. D.: Seasonal variations in the birth of the mentally deficient? *Amer. J. Pub. Health* **50**: 955, 1960.
(6) Medawar, P. B.: *The Art of the Soluble*. London: Methuen, 1967.
(7) Acton, Lord: *A Lecture on the Study of History*. London: Macmillan, 1911.
(8) Pearson, K.: *The Grammar of Science, Part I*. London: Adam and Charles Black, 1911.
(9) de Bono, E.: *The Use of Lateral Thinking*. Harmondsworth: Pelican Books, 1974.
(10) Lakatos, I.: Criticism and the methodology of scientific research programmes. *Proc. Aristotelian Soc.* **69**: 149. 1968.
(11) Yerushalmy, J.: Infants with low birth weight born before their mothers started to smoke cigarettes. *Amer. J. Ob. & Gyn.* **112**: 277, 1972.

168   INTERNATIONAL JOURNAL OF EPIDEMIOLOGY

(12) Anderson, T. W.: Nutritional muscular dystrophy and human myocardial infarction. *Lancet*, **2**: 298, 1973.

(13) Wilson, E. B.: A critical look at statistical epidemiology. *Cancer* **16**: 510, 1963.

(14) Truswell, A. S., Kennelly, B. M., Hansen, J. D. L. and Lee, R. B.: Blood pressures of Kung bushmen in Northern Botswana. *Amer. Heart J.* **84**: 5, 1972.

(15) Poskanzer, D. C., Shapira, K. and Miller, H.: Multiple sclerosis and poliomyelitis. *Lancet* **2**: 917, 1963.

(16) Shekelle, R. B., Ostfeld, A. and Paul, O.: Social status and incidence of coronary heart disease. *J. Chron. Dis.* **22**: 381, 1969.

(17) Neri, L. C., Hewitt, D. and Schreiber, G. B.: Can epidemiology elucidate the water story? *Amer. J. Epid.* **99**: 75, 1974.

(18) Matthews, J. D. and Glasse, R.: Kuru and cannibalism. *Lancet* **2**: 449, 1968.

(19) Snow, J.: *Snow on Cholera—A Reprint of Two Papers.* New York: The Commonwealth Fund, 1936.

(20) Susser: M. *Causal Thinking in the Health Sciences.* New York: Oxford University Press, 1973.

(21) Miettinen, O.: Confounding an effect modification. *Amer. J. Epid.* **100**: 350, 1974.

(22) Fliess, J. L.: *Statistical Methods for Rates and Proportions.* New York: John Wiley, 1973.

(23) MacMahon, B. and Pugh, T. F.: *Epidemiology, Principles and Methods.* Boston: Little, Brown & Co., 1970.

(24) Birtchnell, J.: Is there a scientifically acceptable alternative to the epidemiological study of familial factors in mental illness? *Soc. Sci. & Med.* **8**: 335, 1974.

(25) Cassel, J.: Psychosocial processes and 'stress': theoretical formulation. *Int. J. Health Services* **4**: 471, 1974.

(26) Kennaway, E. L.: The racial and social incidence of cancer of the uterus. *Brit. J. Cancer* **2**: 177, 1948.

(27) Rawls, W. E., Tompkins, W. A. F., Figueroa, M. E. and Melnick, J. L.: Herpesvirus Type 2: Association with carcinoma of the cervix. *Science* **161**: 1255, 1968.

(28) Terris, M.: The relationship of coitus to carcinoma of the cervix. *Amer. J. Pub. Health* **57**: 840, 1967.

(29) Martin, C. E.: Marital and coital factors in cervical cancer. *Amer. J. Pub. Health* **57**: 803, 1967.

(30) Stewart, H. L., Dunham, L. J., Caspar, J., Dorn, H. F., Thomas, L. B., Edgcomb, J. H. and Symeonidis, A.: Epidemiology of cancers of uterine cervix and corpus, breast and ovary in Israel and New York City. *J. Natl. Ca. Inst.* **37**: 1, 1966.

(31) Levitan, M. and Montagu A.: *A Textbook of Human Genetics.* New York: Oxford University Press, 1971.

(32) Pridan, H. and Lilienfeld, A. M.: Carcinoma of the cervix in Jewish women in Israel, 1960–67. *Israeli J. Med. Sci.* **7**(2): 1465, 1971.

(33) Rotkin, I. D.: A comparison review of key epidemiological studies in cervical cancer related to current searches for transmissible agents. *Cancer Res.* **33**: 1353, 1973.

(received 7 April 1975)

International Journal of Epidemiology
© Oxford University Press 1975

Vol. 4, No. 3
Printed in Great Britain

Epidemiological Reasoning

Comments on 'Popper's Philosophy for Epidemiologists' by Carol Buck

COMMENT ONE

> Lest thou make a covenant with the
> inhabitants of the land, and they go a
> whoring after their gods,   *Exodus* 34:15

> And we are right, I think you'll say,
> To argue in this kind of way,
> And I am right
> And you are right
> And all is right—too-looral-lay!
>   W. S. Gilbert: *The Mikado, Act I* (1885)

The two quotations summarize my reactions to Dr. Carol Buck's stimulating paper on 'Popper's philosophy for epidemiologists'. There would be little disagreement as to the desirability of enriching the scope and discipline of epidemiology by applying the ideas of several of the philosophers of science. On the other hand, might there not be a danger of rigidity, of too strict an application of principles derived from the exact sciences to the detriment of the broad development of our discipline? In the present case, why pick on Popper? To play down inductive reasoning and to demote the value of forming hypotheses based on observation could be detrimental to the art, if not to the science as well. If Carol Buck's intention is to make a plea for stricter scientific methods in epidemiological research (and who would disagree?) are there not sufficient lessons to be learned from the masters of epidemiology themselves?

Karl Popper (1) is not easy to understand although it is generally accepted that 'the first strongly reasoned and fully argued exposition of a hypothetico-deductive system is unquestionably Karl Popper's' (2). Dr. Buck agrees with this but, as she also points out, the importance of attempting tests of disproof of hypotheses was already stressed by several of his forebears. Susser (3) paraphrases

Sir Francis Bacon, whose system of inference in science was published in 1559, as 'in other words, the most cogent test of a hypothesis available to scientists is to attempt disproof', citing Popper and Platt (4) in support. Whewell (quoted by Medawar (2)) wrote, as his ninth aphorism in 1840:

> 'The truth of tentative hypotheses must be tested by their application to facts. The discoverer must be ready, carefully to try his hypotheses in this manner . . . and to reject them if they will not bear the test.'

Other forebears, including Lord Acton, Karl Pearson, de Bono and Sherlock Holmes are quoted in Dr. Buck's paper.

Perhaps *the* classics of epidemiology are the two papers of John Snow, reprinted in 1936 (5), where, in his studies on cholera, the author formed a hypothesis, repeatedly tested it and systematically searched for exceptions such as cases who resided away from Broad Street. Thus, he recorded cases in children and adults who were exposed during their school or working hours and noted the absence of cases among brewery workers. In this search for exceptions, Snow anticipated Popper by 100 years. Snow himself was preceded by Sir George Baker, whose 1767 classic on the endemic abdominal colic of Devonshire deserves to be better known (6). At the time, the current hypothesis was that this condition was due to excessive consumption of tartaric acid in apple cider. Supporting evidence was adduced from the existence of a similar condition in the West Indies ascribed to excessive intake of lemon juice. Further 'proof' was the fact that 'precisely the same disease' had been described in 1617 in Poitiers in France among heavy drinkers of the local acid wine.

But, stated Baker, unless the 'colic of Poitou' (Poitiers) was also produced by Rhine and Moselle wines, the analogy does not hold. Was this not seek-

169

2

ing a refutation of the hypothesis? Moreover Turks who drank large quantities of acid sherbert and jockeys who drank much vinegar to lose weight, did not suffer from the colic. The cause could not be consumption of acids.

Nor could it be the cider itself, as inhabitants of other counties of England also drank large quantities of cider but did not have the colic, except on occasion. The clue came from the serendipitous discovery of the fact that in Wurtemberg, adulteration of wine with litharge led to widespread colic while drinking of unadulterated, very acid, wine did not. The symptoms of colic were similar to those suffered by lead workers and an outbreak had occurred in Worcester in those who drank cider which had been stored temporarily in a lead cistern. Note the formation of a new hypothesis based on inductive reasoning and the use of 'natural' experiments to test it.

Finally, Baker proposed the theories that the Devonshire colic was due to lead contamination of the cider and that cider must be prepared differently in Devonshire than in other counties. The former theory he proved by laboratory demonstration of the presence of lead in cider and the latter by examining cider presses and showing that in Devonshire lead was more commonly used to line them or to repair them when cracked.

In Baker's study therefore we have the basic elements of the scientific method as applied to epidemiology. Formation of hypotheses by observation and inductive reasoning: testing by deduction and experiment.

Two hundred years later, Yerushalmy (7) was pointing out that the first requirement for epidemiological studies seeking causal associations is that *all* groups or a random sample of the groups be included, not only those which support the hypothesis. He recalled that the lack of correlation between dietary fat intake and coronary heart disease in certain African tribes and Eskimos, which did not support current hypotheses, was ignored. Yerushalmy's observations on maternal smoking habits and low birthweight, quoted by Carol Buck, have never been satisfactorily explained, although many attempts have been made to dismiss them.

One explanation for our unwillingness to face up to aberrant results is suggested by another philosopher of science, Gerald Holton (8). As Merton puts it in a discussion of Holton's concept:

'The themata of scientific knowledge are tacit cognitive imageries and preferences for or

commitments to certain kinds of concepts, certain kinds of methods, certain kinds of evidence and certain forms of solutions to deep questions and engaging puzzles. Implicit . . . is the notion that they are unevenly accessible to observation' (9).

In Holton's definition, based, according to Merton, on inductive reasoning, there are underlying elements in the concepts, methods and hypotheses of scientific work that function as themes that motivate or constrain the scientist and consolidate or the cognitive judgements appearing in the community of scientists.

But all this has been well stated, in a form relevant to epidemiology, by Susser in a recent book (3); a book that should be required reading for all students and practitioners of the discipline.

At this point, I should state that I benefited greatly from 'Popper's philosophy for epidemiologists' and support Dr. Carol Buck's plea for focusing on the exclusion of hypotheses. But this should only be part of our armamentarium: we must retain inductive methods of reasoning along with deductive methods. Consider the need for imagination and the search for generalization as expressed by Einstein:

'There is no logical way to the discovery of the elemental laws. There is only the way of intuition, which is helped by a feeling for the order lying behind the appearance' (10).

Finally, while we must never forget the need for the strict application of scientific method to epidemiology, we may recall the advice given by Merton to his students.

' "*In general*, it's a good thing to know what you are doing and why you are doing it." The qualifier "in general" is designed, of course, to warn against the danger of that premature fault finding which stifles ideas that need to be played with before being subjected to systematic and rigorous examination. There is a place, as Max Delbruck and Dickinson Richards have severally reminded us, for "the principle of limited sloppiness" '.

A. MICHAEL DAVIES.

Department of Medical Ecology,
Hebrew University,
Hadassah Medical School,
P. O. Box 1172,
Jerusalem, Israel.

POPPER'S PHILOSOPHY FOR EPIDEMIOLOGISTS   171

REFERENCES

(1) Popper, K. R.: *The Logic of Scientific Discovery*. New York: Basic Books, 1959 (reprint of the 1935 edition).

(2) Medawar, P. B.: *The Art of the Soluble*. Harmondsworth: Pelican Books, 1969.

(3) Susser, M.: *Causal Thinking in the Health Sciences*. London: Oxford University Press, 1973.

(4) Platt, J. R.: Strong inference. *Science* 146: 347, 1964.

(5) Snow, J.: *Snow on Cholera, being a reprint of two papers by John Snow, M.D. together with a biographical memoir by B. W. Richardson, M.D. and an introduction by Wade Hampton Frost, M.D.* New York: The Commonwealth Fund. 1936.

(6) Baker, G.: *An Essay Concerning the Cause of the Endemial Colic of Devonshire*. New York: Reprinted by the Delta Omega Society, 1958.

(7) Yerushalmy, J.: On inferring causality from observed associations. In *Controversy in Medicine* (eds. Ingelfinger, Relman and Finland), pp. 659–68. New York: Saunders, 1966.

(8) Holton, G.: *Thematic Origins of Scientific Thought. Kepler to Einstein*. Cambridge, Mass.: Harvard University Press, 1973.

(9) Merton, R. K.: Thematic analysis in science: notes on Holton' concept. *Science* 188: 335, 1975.

(10) Einstein, A., cited by W. I. B. Beveridge: *The Art of Scientific Investigation*, p. 57. London: Mercury Books, 1961.

COMMENT TWO

Whether or not one can accept Dr. Buck's implied thesis that Popper represents the last word in scientific philosophy, her paper is a crucially important contribution to the epidemiological literature. The most important reason why this is so, is that she rejects wholeheartedly the restrictive view of epidemiology that it is primarily concerned with data gathering. Too many epidemiologists have accepted the view that epidemiology is not a domain of enquiry but simply an assembly of methods capable of application to a wide range of medical problems. This view is not only depressing to the would-be epidemiologist but also naive in its implied assumption that the methods of epidemiology are specifically characteristic of that science. They are, of course, the relevant methods of almost any science that is concerned with the study of aspects of human populations.

I like to define epidemiology as the branch of medical science that is concerned to study the health of human communities just as community medicine (or public health in the old nomenclature) is the branch of medical practice that is concerned to promote the health of human communities. Since medicine is a profession and not a trade it is incumbent upon its practitioners to contribute to its science, and upon its scientists to accept some responsibility for its practice. Thus, epidemiology, as the science upon which community medicine practice is based, must seek to provide the body of understanding necessary before decisions in the field of community medicine practice can be other than arbitrary. The epidemiologist must therefore commit himself to explanations that help the practitioners rather than to the illusory pursuit of 'truth' which, if he is honest, results in a perpetual unhelpful agnosticism.

The explanatory function of epidemiology rests, like that of any other science, not upon its body of data but on the set of hypotheses that have survived serious attempts to refute them by data. The explanatory power of such a set of hypotheses depends not only on the rigour of the data testing that they have survived but even more importantly on their mutual coherence. If the set of surviving hypotheses exhibit a high degree of interrelatedness they may be thought of as a body of theory. All well established sciences have such a body of theory out of which new hypotheses arise which lead to purposeful data gathering in the attempt to refute them. If the body of theory is coherent and consistent it may provide a powerful guide to decision and action for practitioners of related fields of professional practice. Thus, for example, we may diagnose and prognose, in clinical medicine, with a confidence based on a body of general understanding of disease processes. In the nineteenth century practitioners of public health (who were usually also practising epidemiologists) could base their recommendations for general environmental hygiene on a general theory of the communicability of diseases without the need to repeat field studies in each locality and on each occasion that a general measure was contemplated. We lack such a body of general theory relating to the important disease problems of today.

Karl Popper's contribution to science—and now specifically to epidemiology by the good offices of Dr. Buck—has been to stress that data and the methodology of their collection represent the ordeal through which hypotheses must pass before being admitted to the status of theory, and that it is theory and not data that is the functional element in science. Epidemiology, like any other science, therefore depends not on its data and not on the elaboration of its methodology but on the thought that goes into erecting the hypotheses whose surviving fraction will eventually constitute the central understanding which alone can justify a science.

ALWYN SMITH.

Department of Preventive and Social Medicine,
Clinical Sciences Building,
York Place,
Manchester, M13 OHH, England.

Popper's Philosophy for Epidemiologists

From Mr. Andrew Creese:

SIR—I feel that the Comments on *Popper's Philosophy for Epidemiologists* (*Int. J. Epid.* 1975, *4*: 169) rather fail to do credit to the case against Popper's concept of scientific progress. Among philosophers of science, the debate about and around Popper has been long and deep (1), and though I cannot attempt to summarize it I should like to raise three points arising from it which are relevant to Dr. Buck's transfer of Popperian method to epidemiology.

First, the advance of scientific knowledge does not occur in a historical, social or political vacuum, as one might assume from Dr. Buck's interpretation. Popperian science is not value free, if by this we mean that hypotheses can be conceived independently of the individual values of the investigator, the professional values of a particular branch of science, or some broader social preference. In what has been interpreted as an alternative view of scientific progress, Thomas Kuhn (2) has argued that scientific communities in particular subscribe to a common paradigm or pattern, in accordance with which 'normal' scientific research identifies the appropriate hypotheses to test, and the appropriate conclusions to draw from their falsification. The paradigm varies between sciences, but broadly it can be understood as a loose model of the 'real' universe, of sufficient cohesiveness to indicate to scientists where the needs for research are most urgent. Conversely, and importantly, the paradigm also suggests where research is unnecessary or unlikely to be fruitful. The paradigm is promoted through textbooks and articulated in scientific practice, and it is by reference to it that bad science can be identified. A dramatic illustration of such a thought convention is the pre-Copernican paradigm of celestial order. It is the paradigms of normal science, like the germ theory of disease, which are the most powerful obstacles to imaginative thought, and not the individual hypotheses themselves as Dr. Buck claims, and the paradigms are complex fabrics of accumulated knowledge, habit, and modes of perception. Two quotations from Kuhn are appropriate:

> *For a scientist, the solution of a difficult conceptual or instrumental puzzle is a principal goal. His success in that endeavour is rewarded through recognition by other members of his professional group and by them alone. The practical merit of his solution is at best a secondary value, and the*

approval of men outside the specialist group is a negative value or none at all. These values, which do much to dictate the form of normal science, are also significant when a choice must be made between theories.

The professional paradigm thus channels our potential for lateral thought, and an understanding of the sociological and psychological influences on scientific progress should be part of the philosophy of scientific knowledge:

Already it should be clear that the explanation must, in the final analysis, be psychological or sociological. It must, that is, be a description of a value system, an ideology, together with an analysis of the institutions through which that system is transmitted and enforced. Knowing what scientists value, we may hope to understand what problems they will undertake and what choices they will make in particular circumstances of conflict (3).

The notion of cultural conditioning of scientific progress leads to my second point: the value and purpose of scientific enquiry. Popper's advice on hypothesis generating is appropriate as a workshop manual—in fact it is the highest statement of the technique, and Dr. Buck is right to place her article in the context of 'an impending withdrawal of the *carte blanche* that for so long has been offered to science'. But we are again at the level of daily practice, or action, which Dr. Buck appreciates is a poor source of productive habits of thought. Does science have a social purpose or even incidentally a social value? Popperian method gives no indication, since it attempts to perfect a logic of knowledge without reference to the sociocultural background, or even to the psychology of the scientific group. As long as we are prepared to postpone a concern with the meaning of scientific discovery Popper is an infallible guide; but as soon as we ask for a foothold in contemporary problems, the gap between scientific knowledge and social concern becomes clear. We are surely entitled to expect the philosophers of science to consider the relationship between science and society.

Thirdly, and again continuing from the previous point, it really is necessary to be aware of Popper's

own political stance to comprehend his pursuit of objectivity in the description and prescription of scientific method. That he has a political aim is clear—in fact Kuhn suggests that Popper presents an ideology, not a logic, of scientific discovery. Popper is a political pragmatist, as is evident from *The Poverty of Historicism* (4), and his approach to social problems is one of piecemeal intervention rather than wholesale change. Essentially conservative, therefore, his method of investigation is one of tinkering at the edges (witness the test of hypotheses) rather than attempting to assess the process by which the conceptual categories which structure our selection of problems and our perception of them are formed. Hypotheses are the result of a process of conceptual categorization which is itself worth analysing, and which certainly involves interaction between the individual and his environment. What we have to ask to extend the scope of scientific knowledge is thus not whether a particular hypothesis satisfies Popper's standards, or what are the possible alternatives, but what are the relevant influences on scientific perception?

We may not, on a daily basis, need to be aware of the wider factors shaping particular areas of experimentation, nor of the extent and nature of the relationship of science and the community. Popper's prescriptions are then sound practical and professional advice. But this should not be confused with a philosophy of what are, arguably, the more important questions facing science in general and epidemiology in particular.

REFERENCES

(1) Lakatos, I. and Musgrave, A. (Eds.): *Criticism and the Growth of Knowledge.* Cambridge University Press, 1970.
(2) Kuhn, T. S.: *The Structure of Scientific Revolutions.* University of Chicago Press, 1962.
(3) Kuhn, T. S.: in (1).
(4) Popper, K.: *The Poverty of Historicism.* Routledge and Kegan Paul, 1957.

Lecturer in Health Economics,
Department of Social Administration,
London School of Economics,
Houghton Street,
London, WC2.   *30 October 1975*

International Journal of Epidemiology
© Oxford University Press 1976

Vol. 5, No. 1
Printed in Great Britain

Letters to the Editor

Cervical cancer and early sexual intercourse

From Mr. Richard Peto:

SIR—Dr. Buck (1) considers various explanations for the relevance of early exposure to sexual intercourse to subsequent incidence rates of cervical cancer. All these explanations invoke some putative special susceptibility of the adolescent cervix. However, early exposure would be expected to be very relevant even if no such special susceptibility existed.

Suppose an organ (the cervix, in this case) is exposed for a certain amount of time to a repeated carcinogenic insult. After a number of years of such treatment have passed, there is an appreciable probability that a pathological cancer will appear in that organ in the coming year. The point to note is that this probability (the 'incidence rate' of pathological cancer) increases very sharply with duration of exposure to the insult; for example, with lung cancer, where the start of the insult can be timed, incidence rates increase roughly as the fourth power of duration of smoking, but *given* this duration the age of the subject doesn't matter. This strong relationship with duration of insult can, however, give the mistaken impression that some special susceptibility of the young must be invoked. Again, consider lung cancer incidence rates after various durations of smoking. Among men who smoke one pack of cigarettes a day from the age of 20 for the rest of their lives, the risk of lung cancer in their 40th year of smoking will be about three times as big as the risk in their 30th year of smoking (since $40^4/30^4 \simeq 3$). This isn't because ageing itself matters, it's just because the duration of past smoking is longer in the older men. An exactly equivalent observation would be to note that in a group of regular smokers of one pack per day who are all aged 55, those who started to smoke at 15 had an incidence rate of lung cancer three times greater than that of the men who started smoking at 25. Smoking between the ages of 15 and 25 thus triples the risk at 55, and this might misleadingly suggest that young adult lungs are especially vulnerable, while in fact the exact opposite is true—the effects of cigarette smoke on the lung tissue of regular smokers depend only on duration of exposure and, given this, are wholly independent of the age at which the exposure occurs.

This is found in both experimental animals and humans (2) and so one would expect, for example, to find (if the adolescent cervix is no more vulnerable than the adult cervix) that women of 40 who started intercourse at 15 have more than twice the incidence rate of cervical among otherwise similar women who only started intercourse at 20.

The age distribution of cervical cancer is, in middle and old age, complicated by the effects of age-related changes in sexual habits as well as, perhaps, by some genuine age-related changes at the menopause. Nevertheless, the *necessary* strong relationship between the age when intercourse begins and subsequent risk should be recognized in any interpretation of the *observed* relationship between these factors, even if, as in Professor Buck's article, this interpretation is merely a teaching example.

REFERENCES

(1) Buck, Carol. *International Journal of Epidemiology*, **4**, 159, 1975.
(2) Peto, R., *et al. British Journal of Cancer*, **32**, 411, 1975.

Department of the Regius Professor of Medicine,
Radcliffe Infirmary,
Oxford, OX2 6HE   *11 November 1975*

Popper's Philosophy for Epidemiologists

From Dr. Carol Buck:

SIR—I am indebted to Michael Davies (1), Alwyn Smith (2), Michael Jacobson (3), Richard Peto (4) and Andrew Creese (5) for taking the trouble to comment on my paper *Popper's Philosophy for Epidemiologists* (6). Being mindful of space limitations, I shall not attempt to reply to all the points that they have made.

Andrew Creese's letter is concerned with *what* scientists investigate, whereas my paper dealt with *how* scientists conduct their investigations. I think he is wrong in suggesting that my article invites the assumption that science advances in a historical and political vacuum. I do not believe this nor did I intend to imply it. I agree with him that scientists have an obligation to direct some of their effort towards society's current problems. But, as Popper has emphasized, a problem cannot be attacked scientifically unless it lends itself to the formulation of testable hypotheses. For this reason some of society's concerns lie at present outside the domain of science, a fact which we may regret but for which we cannot, in my view, blame Popper.

Michael Davies and Michael Jacobsen both chide me for downgrading induction, although in different ways.

Dr. Davies insists on the old prescription: 'formation of hypotheses by observation and inductive reasoning, testing by deduction and experiment'. His chief example is Baker's serendipitous discovery of the relationship between adulterated wine and colic in Wurtemberg. He appears to believe that the occurrence of serendipity destroys Popper's premise that all observations are made to test some hypothesis already in mind. Not everyone believes this, and certainly not Pasteur who said, 'In the fields of observation, chance favours only the mind that is prepared'.

Mr. Jacobson's criticism attacks my implied dismissal of statistics as 'a set of numerical devices'. I am sorry if this is what I implied, because my respect for the contribution of statistics to epidemiology is deep and of long duration. I agree fully with Jacobson that statistical inference is an inductive process indispensable to the interpretation of data and hence to the testing of hypotheses. Moreover, I do not interpret Popper's views as being in conflict with the principles of statistical inference. Popper's point is that induction plays little part in the *generation* of hypotheses.

Mr. Jacobson's paper offers an argument against my expectation of a positive association between habitual abortion and cervical cancer if both are related to a deficiency of progesterone. He demonstrates that unless both of the associations with progesterone are strong, the correlation between abortion and cervical cancer can be zero, or even negative. I am grateful for being appraised of this restriction upon the behaviour of correlations among three random variables.

Richard Peto suggests that a special susceptibility of the adolescent cervix need not be invoked to explain the high relative risk associated with coitus under the age of 17 and that duration of exposure would suffice. It seemed to me that his model would not account for the fact that when age at first coitus is dichotomized at under 20 years versus 20 years and over, the relative risk is almost the same as when the dichotomy is made at 17 years. (I have made these comparisons using data from six studies summarized by Rotkin (7).) My colleague in the Department of Mathematics, Dr. Jon Baskerville, has examined this question. He finds that the lung cancer model, with incidence related to the fourth power of duration of smoking, gives a steep rise in risk ratios as the point of dichotomy is advanced along the age span. However when he postulated a different model, in which incidence increases in simple proportion to the length of exposures, the risk ratios increase so slowly as the point of dichotomy advances that the relative risk for under 20 years versus 20 years and over is only marginally greater than that for under 17 years versus 17 years and over, as in the calculations that I made from Rotkin's data. However, one can achieve the same result from Peto's model by adding to it a special susceptibility under the age of 17. It is unlikely, therefore, that the issue can be settled by an appeal to models. The hypotheses of special susceptibility in adolescence would be refuted if we found that women who started sexual activity at 15 and stopped at 25 had no greater risk of cervical carcinoma than women who started at 20 and stopped at 30. Perhaps we should start looking for some convents that do not require virginity as a condition of entry. This need not be regarded as a completely facetious suggestion if one recalls the epidemiological significance of Gagnon's observation in 1950 on the rarity of cervical cancer among nuns (8).

Since my paper appeared, a friend has told me that I may be wrong in regarding as bizarre the assumption that orthodoxy is equally frequent among New York and Israeli Jews. According to his sources of information, the proportion of observant Jews is thought to be about 30 per cent in both areas.

Department of Epidemiology and Preventive Medicine,
Faculty of Medicine,
The University of Western Ontario,
London, Canada   *26 January 1976*

REFERENCES

(1) Davies, A. Michael. *International Journal of Epidemiology*, **4**: 169, 1975.
(2) Smith, Alwyn. *International Journal of Epidemiology*, **4**: 171, 1975.
(3) Jacobson, M.: *International Journal of Epidemiology* **5**: 9, 1976.
(4) Peto, R. *International Journal of Epidemiology* **5**: 97, 1976.
(5) Creese, A. L.: *International Journal of Epidemiology* **4**: 352, 1975.
(6) Buck, Carol.: *International Journal of Epidemiology* **4**: 159, 1975.
(7) Rotkin, I. D.: *Cancer Research* **33**: 1353, 1973
(8) Gagnon, F.: *American Journal of Obstetrics and Gynecology* **60**: 516, 1950.

International Journal of Epidemiology
© Oxford University Press 1976

Vol. 5, No. 1
Printed in Great Britain

Against Popperized Epidemiology

M. JACOBSEN[1]

Jacobsen, M. (Institute of Occupational Medicine, Roxburgh Place, Edinburgh, EH8 9SU, Scotland). Against Popperized Epidemiology. *International Journal of Epidemiology*. 1976, **5**: 9–11.
The recommendation that Popper's philosophy of science should be adopted by epidemiologists is disputed. Reference is made to other authors who have shown that the most constructive elements in Popper's ideas have been advocated by earlier philosophers and have been used in epidemiology without abandoning inductive reasoning. It is argued that Popper's denigration of inductive methods is particularly harmful to epidemiology. Inductive reasoning and statistical inference play a key role in the science; it is suggested that unfamiliarity with these ideas contributes to widespread misunderstanding of the function of epidemiology. Attention is drawn to a common fallacy involving correlations between three random variables. The prevalence of the fallacy may be related to confusion between deductive and inductive logic.

In a recent paper (1) Dr. Carol Buck protests that epidemiologists should not be regarded, by themselves or by others, as data-gathering adjuncts to the medical-scientific community. She argues that creative epidemiology requires the formulation of refutable hypotheses and that epidemiologists should involve themselves more in the "exciting process of scientific deduction". Her view is that the achievement of these laudable objectives would be promoted if epidemiologists were to adopt the ideas of Karl Popper. Yet Dr. Buck herself and Davies (2) refer to some of Popper's predecessors who understood and emphasized the importance of attempting to refute scientific hypotheses. Dr. Davies asks 'why pick on Popper?'

A major distinguishing feature in Popper's philosophy is his insistence that his ideas are 'directly opposed to all attempts to operate with the ideas of inductive logic' (3). Dr. Buck accepts this view enthusiastically. I agree with Dr. Davies. This is not a helpful way to free epidemiologists from the misunderstanding that their task is merely to 'gather data from which other scientists will build hypotheses' (1). On the contrary, I have argued elsewhere (4) that because good medical practice relies heavily on the deductive art of diagnosis, many physicians appear to have great difficulty in appreciating the rules and discipline of epidemiological research, since here the inductive method of reasoning is paramount. Unfamiliarity with inductive reasoning is one of the barriers obstructing an understanding of the role of statistical

inference in epidemiology; and statistical inference lies at the heart of epidemiology. Why? Because epidemiology is concerned largely with the study of observations which are subject to random fluctuations.

Dr. Buck warns against 'an excessive recourse to statistical devices for tidying up epidemiological data'. It is useful to draw the attention of epidemiologists to Cox's objection to equating statistical inference with data summarization (5). Cox reminds us that in statistical inference 'an essential element is the uncertainty involved in passing from the observations to the underlying population'. In Cox's formulation it is the element of uncertainty which makes the inference statistical; the *direction* of the argument, *from* the observations *to* the (statistical) population sampled, is characteristic of the inductive method. Note that if this inductive step is taken with a proper regard to the logic underlying (for instance) a test of statistical significance (the logic includes its restricted relevance to the population sampled), then the induction leads naturally to what Dr. Buck calls the 'deductively more powerful' reason for replication in epidemiology: to identify circumstances under which a previously observed association does not exist.

In common with some other epidemiologists Dr. Buck appears to regard applied statistics essentially as a set of numerical 'devices'. However, in epidemiology as elsewhere, the application of probability theory to real data embraces more than significance testing, standardization and data summarization. For instance, an increasingly important part of modern epidemiology is directed to determining the relationship between the dose of a suspected or

[1] Institute of Occupational Medicine, Roxburgh Place, Edinburgh EH8 9SU, Scotland.

known environmental pollutant and the degree of response in human populations. The solution to this quantitative problem requires, among other things, statistical point estimation (of the regression coefficient for instance) and interval estimation. The latter may involve controversial inferences about the distribution of the unknown regression coefficient being estimated or the interval containing the estimate itself, at a fixed probability level. The fact that significance testing may be relatively unimportant in such situations, and that it may be difficult to force the pertinent research questions into a formal hypothesis implying a refutable prediction, does not convince me that this activity therefore lies outside the boundary of science. Of course, once the dose-response relationship has been estimated then this provides the basis for subsequent predictions which are refutable in principle. Indeed I have suggested two ways whereby such epidemiologically derived predictions can be tested in practice (6). The important point to note however is that the initial estimation of the dose-response relationship requires inductive arguments of statistical inference, from the sample to the population parameters of interest. Deductions and hypotheses follow.

The discussion in the two preceding paragraphs illustrates Fisher's point that 'deductive arguments are, in fact, often only stages in an inductive process' (7). Popper (3) would be unmoved by these considerations. He distinguishes between inductive processes, which he relegates to the realm 'psychology of knowledge', and the deductive method, which he considers as part of the 'logic of knowledge'. He then asserts that he is concerned only with the latter. ('There is no need even to mention induction.') Even if this view is acceptable to one who is dedicated specifically to the search for a wholly abstract theory of knowledge, it is difficult to see why Dr. Buck commends it to epidemiologists who are involved directly in the practice of an empirical science which leans heavily on inductive methods.

For her 'exercise in Popperian epidemiology' Dr. Buck (1) reformulates the 'infectious hypothesis' concerning cancer of the uterine cervix. Her hypothesis asserts, *inter alia*, a negative correlation between the risk of cervical cancer and progesterone levels. Dr. Buck then proceeds to discuss testable predictions from the hypothesis. One of them states

'A history of repeated spontaneous abortion should be associated with cervical cancer, because susceptibility to abortion is to some extent related to low levels of progesterone.'

This prediction does not follow from the hypothesis (quite apart from the careful caveats made by Dr. Buck herself). Let X, Y and Z represent the random variables of cervical cancer incidence, progesterone level and spontaneous abortion incidence respectively; let r_{XY}, r_{ZY} and r_{XZ} be the correlation coefficients between XY, ZY and XZ. Dr. Buck's prediction can be written as

$$\begin{rcases} \text{'if} \quad r_{XY}<0 \\ \text{and} \quad r_{ZY}<0 \end{rcases} \text{[1]}$$
$$\text{then} \quad r_{XZ}>0\text{'.} \quad\text{[2]}$$

The assertion [2] is a *non-sequitur* not uncommon among epidemiologists. The difficulty seems to be connected with confusion between deductive and inductive methods of argument. Only the simplest algebra or common (deductive) sense suffices to show that

$$\begin{rcases} \text{if} \quad x=a_0+a_1y \\ \text{and} \quad z=b_0+b_1y, \end{rcases} \text{[3]}$$

where x, y and z are real variables; a, b are constants; and a_1, b_1 are non-zero;

$$\text{then} \quad x=c_0+c_1z, \quad\text{[4]}$$

where $c_1=a_1/b_1\neq0$. Moreover, if a_1 and b_1 have the same algebraic sign, then $c_1>0$. Now it is easy to write down linear regression models [5] embodying the left-hand sides of the inequalities [1] and [2], and they look deceptively similar to equations [3] and [4].

$$\begin{rcases} E(X|y)=\alpha_0+\alpha_1y \\ E(Z|y)=\beta_0+\beta_1y \\ E(X|z)=\gamma_0+\gamma_1z \end{rcases} \text{[5]}$$

If α_1 and β_1 are known to be negative it does not follow that γ_1 is positive.

Why is the deductive algebraic syllogism of [3] and [4] not applicable to the models [5]? Because the models refer to *random* systems; they are not simple linear equations. The coefficient γ_1 is an unknown population parameter. It may be estimated from appropriate data using inductive, statistical arguments. The degree of uncertainty in the estimate would be related to the variance of the random variable X. (In reality, we cannot 'know' that α_1 and β_1 are both negative; but, given enough data, and using inductive arguments, we may have great confidence that this is true.)

The argument from [1] to [2] is false; but it can

AGAINST POPPERIZED EPIDEMIOLOGY   **11**

be shown that there are conditions constraining r_{xz} to be positive when r_{xy} and r_{zy} have the same algebraic sign. The inequalities

$$1 > r_{xy} r_{zy} > 0 \qquad\qquad [6]$$
$$r_{xy} r_{zy} - [(r_{xy}^2 - 1)(r_{zy}^2 - 1)]^{\frac{1}{2}} > 0 \qquad [7]$$

are sufficient conditions to satisfy [2]. The necessary condition for $r_{xz} \leqslant 0$, given [6], is that the left-hand side of [7] $\leqslant 0$. Thus if r_{xy} and r_{zy} both exceed $+\sqrt{0\cdot 5} \approx 0\cdot 71$ (or are both less than $-0\cdot 71$) then $r_{xz} > 0$. However, there may be a wide range of paired values (r_{xy}, r_{zy}) with the same algebraic sign and $r_{xz} \leqslant 0$. For example, if $r_{xy} = -0\cdot 8$ and $r_{zy} = -0\cdot 4$, then non-positive values of r_{xz} may be as low as $-0\cdot 2299$; certainly r_{xz} may be zero. Or, if $r_{xy} = r_{zy} = 0\cdot 5$, then r_{xz} may be as low as $-0\cdot 5$.

For those who prefer a non-theoretical refutation of the assertion hypothesising that 'the inequality [2] follows logically from [1]' it is sufficient to find any data set where the assertion is contradicted. The contrived data below meet the purpose.

x	y	z
0	4	6
1	5	1
2	0	4
4	6	2
5	1	5
6	2	0

$r_{xy} = r_{zy} = -0\cdot 29; \; r_{xz} = -0\cdot 43.$

Fisher (7) has remarked on a 'tendency to impose on inductive thought the conventions and preconceptions appropriate only to deductive reasoning.' Popper states (3): *'Believers in probability logic may try to meet my criticism'* (of inductive methods) *'by asserting that it springs from a mentality which is "tied to the framework of classical logic", and which is therefore incapable of following the methods of reasoning employed by probability logic. I freely admit that I am incapable of following these methods of reasoning.'* The concluding admission is deplorable even if it was intended facetiously.

I agree with Dr. Buck that epidemiology would benefit if more of the data gathering were preceded by the formulation of hypotheses whose relevance to science will have been deduced from previously established knowledge. The element of deduction in the formulation of the hypotheses does not make induction irrelevant, any more than the essential inductive inferences from observed data negate the importance of prior and subsequent deductions.

REFERENCES

(1) Buck, C.: Popper's philosophy for epidemiologists. *International Journal of Epidemiology* 4: 159, 1975.
(2) Davies, A. M.: Comments on 'Popper's philosophy for epidemiologists' by Carol Buck. *International Journal of Epidemiology* 4: 169, 1975.
(3) Popper, K. R.: *The Logic of Scientific Discovery.* Sixth impression (revised), pp. 30, 315, 265. London: Hutchinson, 1972.
(4) Jacobsen, M.: A science which ought to be honourable. *Transactions of the Society of Occupational Medicine* 21: 38, 1971.
(5) Cox, D. R.: Some problems connected with statistical inference. *Annals of Mathematical Statistics* 29: 357, 1958.
(6) Jacobsen, M.: Evidence of dose-response relation in pneumoconiosis (2). *Transactions of the Society of Occupational Medicine* 22: 88, 1972.
(7) Fisher, R. A.: *Statistical Methods and Scientific Inference.* Second edition, pp. 109, 110. Edinburgh: Oliver and Boyd, 1959.

I–9.

Mervyn Susser: Judgment and Causal Inference:
Criteria in Epidemiologic Studies.
American Journal of Epidemiology 1977; 105:1–15.

Susser's "Judgment and Causal Inference: Criteria in Epidemiologic Studies" contains a message that I suspect will continue to require reinforcement for decades to come: that causal inference should not be equated with statistical inference, and in particular that statistical expertise alone is insufficient for causal analysis of data. Susser brought this message home not by abstract arguments, but by fascinating historical illustrations of how failure to appreciate the nonstatistical aspects of causal inference led to major inferential errors by renowned statisticians. The last paragraph of Susser's quote from Wright (p.5) illustrates an early awareness of the predominant importance of nonstatistical sources of error, such as confounding ("want of conformity between the test cases and control cases") and misclassification.

Susser argued that overreliance on statistical criteria tends to lead to excessive false-negative judgments regarding causality. Some of the conservative bias observed by Susser may be attributed not to overemphasis of statistics *per se,* but rather an overreliance on certain statistical methods, especially significance testing [Rothman, 1978 and 1986; Salsburg, 1985; Wonnacott, 1985; Gardner and Altman, 1986]. Empirical evidence for such "test-based" bias has been given by Freiman et al., [1978]. But all statistical methods are limited to dealing with precisely quantified sources of error. When unquantified sources of error are recognizably the largest ones, Susser argued that judgment must take precedence over statistical inference.

One can also see in Susser's examples the tension between the scientific and public-health objectives of epidemiologic research. As scientists, epidemiologists (and statisticians) may be well-advised to adopt a Popperian attitude and never treat a causal explanation of an association as anything more than a tentative hypothesis about nature. While a pure scientist can always afford to wait for more evidence to test such explanations, a fair number of epidemiologists are health officials or close advisors of executive authorities, and will be confronted with situations demanding action. Susser recognized that the latter situations require principles beyond those of statistical and causal inference, and that these principles need to be elucidated by and for such epidemiologists, much as principles of statistical and causal inference have been elucidated by earlier authors.

References:
Freiman JA, Chalmers TC, Smith H, et al. The importance of beta, the Type II error and sample size in the design and interpretation of the randomized control data. N Engl J Med 1978; 299:690–694.
Gardner MJ, Altman DG. Confidence intervals rather than P values: estimation rather than testing. Br Med J 1986; 292:746–750.
Rothman KJ. A show of confidence. N Engl J Med 1978; 299:1362–1363.
Rothman KJ. *Modern Epidemiology.* Boston: Little, Brown, 1986.
Salsburg DS. The religion of statistics as practiced by medical journals. Am Statist 1985; 39:220–223.
Wonnacott T. "Statistically significant." Can Med Assoc J 1985; 133:843.

JUDGMENT AND CAUSAL INFERENCE: CRITERIA IN EPIDEMIOLOGIC STUDIES

MERVYN SUSSER

The processes of statistical inference, those of causal inference, and those of reaching decisions often overlap, but the principles that govern them are not the same (1). Clinicians, epidemiologists and applied statisticians often experience a tension between the formal requirements of a statistical test of a result on the one hand, and the practical requirements of a judgment about the application of the result on the other. Formal statistical tests are framed to give mathematical answers to structured questions leading to judgments, whereas in any field practitioners must give answers to unstructured questions leading from judgment to decision and implementation. These questions of decision generally hinge around judgments about causality and prediction (2). Once-famous historical controversies will serve to illuminate them. The approach is thus that of the case-history and not of the epidemiologic survey, with all the selectiv-

ity the method implies. Nonetheless, from our position of after-knowledge, we have the advantage of observing major figures exercising their judgments as part of the historical evolution of decisions of which we know the consequences.

An early illustration of a statistician's mathematical answer to a structured question is William Farr's formula, the first for an epidemic curve. Farr, a physician appointed as the Compiler of Statistical Abstracts of the newly-founded General Register Office in London in 1839, analyzed the data for the smallpox epidemic of 1837–1839 to show how the disease regularly rose to a peak and declined (3, 4). He then calculated the equivalent of a normal frequency curve and showed that it fitted the observed frequencies of smallpox deaths by quarter-year (5, 6). Exhibit 1 is taken from Farr's report.

An illustration, some 25 years later, of an epidemiologist making a judgment about a practical question is again provided by William Farr, in a letter to the London *Daily News* of February 17, 1866 about the raging and unfamiliar rinderpest epidemic among cattle (6). As mortality among animals continued on a sharply rising curve, the Right Honourable Robert Lowe, a major figure in the parliamentary

From the Division of Epidemiology, Columbia University School of Public Health, 600 W. 168th. St., New York, NY 10032.

Read at the meeting of the Biometrics Society, St. Paul, MN, March 25, 1975.

The author acknowledges the contributions to the development of this paper made by Drs. Agnes Berger, Joseph Fleiss and Zena Stein, as well as by several members of his seminar classes.

1

2   MERVYN SUSSER

EXHIBIT 1

Extracts from William Farr's letter to the Registrar General, Second Annual Report of the Registrar General,
1840 (from Humphreys NA (ed.): Vital Statistics: A Memorial Volume of the Reports and Writings of William
Farr. London, Sanitary Institute of Great Britain, 1885, pp. 318-319 (reference 4))

	Small-Pox									
	1837		1838					1839		
Periods	1	2	3	4	5	6	7	8	9	10
Seasons	Summer	Autumn	Winter	Spring	Summer	Autumn	Winter	Spring	Summer	Autumn
Deaths	2513	3289	4242	4489	3685	3851	2982	2505	1533	1730

If the latent cause of epidemics cannot be discovered, the mode in which it operates
may be investigated. The laws of its action may be determined by observation, as well
as the circumstances in which epidemics arise, or by which they may be controlled.

Amidst the apparent irregularities of the epidemic of small-pox, and its eruptions all
over the kingdom, it was governed in its progress by certain general laws. The deaths
in the early stage of the epidemic were not registered. To avoid circumlocution, it will
be convenient to call the ten quarters in which the deaths were registered the ten
periods, the first quarter the first period, the second the second period, etc., etc. The
mortality increased up to the fourth registered period; the deaths in the first were 2513,
in the second 3289, in the third 4242; and it will be perceived at a glance that these
numbers increased very nearly at the rate of 30 per cent. For multiply 2513 by 1.30 and
it will become 3267; multiply 3267 by 1.30 and it will become 4248. The rate of increase is
retarded at the end of the third period, and only rises 6 per cent in the next, where it
remains stationary, like a projectile at the summit of the curve which it is destined to
describe.

The decline of the epidemic was less rapid than its rise, and the mortality was
somewhat greater in the autumns of 1838 and 1839 than in the summers. But by taking
the mean of the deaths in the third and fourth period, the mean of the deaths in the
fourth and fifth period, etc., etc., a regular series of numbers is produced.

Deaths observed in the decline of the Epidemic

1	2	3	4	5	6	7
4365	4087	3767	3416	2743	2019	1631

Deaths in regular series

1	2	3	4	5	6	7
4364	4147	3767	3272	2716	2156	1635

The 4365 may be considered to represent the deaths that happened between the
middle of February and the middle of May. The regular series of numbers has been
calculated upon the hypothesis that the fall of the mortality took place at a uniformly
accelerated rate.

The calculated numbers are sometimes a little too high, and sometimes too low; but,
on the whole, the agreement is remarkable. The second number (4147) is nearly 5 per
cent lower than the first; and the decrease is successively 5, 10, 15, 20, 26, and 32 per
cent. The rates of decrease are 1.052, 1.101, 1.152, 1.205, 1.260, 1.318. The division of
4364 by 1.052 reduces it to 4147; the division of 4147 by 1.101 produces 3767, etc. The
mortality decreased at accelerated rates; and the rate of acceleration was 1.046, which,
by successive multiplication, will reproduce all the rates, 1.052, 1.101, etc., etc. The rate
1.046 may be called the constant.

opposition, announced impending national doom. Mr. Lowe's argument was that " . . . there is no reason why the same terrible law of increase which has prevailed hitherto should not prevail henceforth." Farr, even though he was a longtime civil servant, did not hesitate to confute Mr. Lowe in the press. "No one," he wrote, "can express a proposition more clearly than Mr. Lowe but the clearness of a proposition is no evidence of its truth." Previous experience of epidemics, Farr argued, showed that the alarm was false, and that a decline from the peak would soon follow. He made his prediction of a downturn merely on the basis of a series of four 4-week averages of mortality. Nothing but judgment founded on his 30-year experience could have allowed Farr to venture so much on so little, and his prediction, although a little optimistic, was soon confirmed (see Exhibit 2).

In another such controversy that I will use as an example, the protagonists, Karl Pearson and Almroth Wright, were more evenly matched. In 1896 Wright had developed a vaccine against typhoid (more or less at the same time as Pfeiffer) (7). Wright's vaccine had been tried out among volunteers in the British Army first in India and later in the South African war (8). In 1904 a specially appointed Committee of the Medical Advisory Board to the War Office, including Wright, recommended on the basis of the data collected by these means that the Army adopt routine inoculation against typhoid.

The Medical Advisory Board referred the Committee's report to Professor Pearson (who, Wright said, was a Rhadamanthys to whom all inoculators must come to have judgment passed). Pearson's review of the data was published in the *British Medical Journal* of November 5, 1904 (9). He separately analyzed the data for incidence (these came from five sources) and for case-fatality (these came from six). In each case, he calculated a (tetrachoric) coefficient of correlation.

Pearson appreciated the insufficiency of statistical significance alone for making decisions. In advance of his analysis, he ingeniously derived a judgmental criterion from the available experience with smallpox and diphtheria inoculation, both of which were by then in use. Pearson decided that with a correlation coefficient of 0.6 or more, as with smallpox, the new procedure would be clearly justified; he noted that even with a coefficient between 0.24 and 0.47, as with diphtheria antitoxin treatment, the procedure had been "universally" adopted by the medical profession, and the typhoid vaccine could be recommended above this level.

The results were as follows (Exhibit 3): In all but two of the eleven instances (IV and VII on the table), "the correlations were at least twice, and generally four, five, or more times their probable errors", and hence statistically significant by Pearson's own criterion. But the mean value of the correlations fell below the acceptable preset level ("0.2 or even 0.3"). Unlike smallpox vaccination, wrote Pearson, the effect of typhoid inoculation was inconsistent: in his words, "largely influenced by differences of environment or of treatment," and he did not think the results yielded a pattern sufficiently coherent to be trustworthy.* He recommended further investigation and prophylactic trials, and the suspension of inoculation as a routine measure. He wrote further that "if it were not presumption . . . I should say that the data indicate a more effective serum or effective method of administration must be found before inoculation ought to become a routine practice . . . "

Wright responded to Pearson's report, and an accompanying editorial in the *British Medical Journal*, with a tirade (10,

---

* Both Pearson and Wright were aware of the problems of using volunteers, in terms of self-selection and comparability with controls. Pearson thought that the caution of volunteers for vaccination may have accounted for the variation in the South African results between immobile and mobile troops.

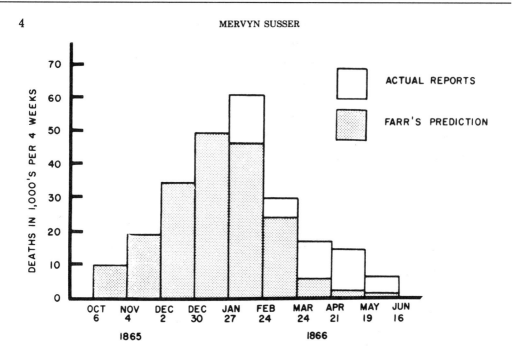

Periods of Four Weeks ending	Reported Attacks	Calculated Series by "Law"	Actual Figures
1865			
November 4	9,597		
December 2	18,817		
December 30	33,835		
1866			
January 27	47,191		
February 24		43,182	57,004
March 24		21,927	27,958
April 21		5,228	15,856
May 19		494	14,734
June 16		16	5,000 (about)

EXHIBIT 2. Epizootic cattle plague (rinderpest) epidemic, London, October 1865 to June 1866. (Data taken from Langmuir A: The role of William Farr in the development of the concept of surveillance (unpublished paper).)

JUDGMENT AND CAUSAL INFERENCE   5

EXHIBIT 3*

Inoculation against enteric fever

	Inoculated			Non-inoculated			Immunity and Inoculation		Odds Ratios
	No.	Cases	Deaths	No.	Cases	Deaths	r	P.E.	
I. Hospital Staffs	297	32	2	279	75	12	.373 ± .021		3.04
II. Ladysmith Garrison	1,705	35	8	10,529	1,489	329	.445 ± .017		7.86
III. Methuen's Column	2,535	26	?	10,981	257	?	.191 ± .026		2.31
IV. Single Regiments	1,207	72	9	1,285	82	21	.021 ± .033		1.07
V. Army in India	15,389	128	20	136,360	2,132	569	.100 ± .013		1.74
Mean Value							.226		

	Recoveries	Deaths	Recoveries	Deaths	Case Fatality and Inoculation		Odds Ratios
					r	P.E.	
VI. Hospital Staffs	30	2	63	12	.307 ± .128		2.86
VII. Ladysmith Garrison	27	8	1,160	329	−.010 ± .081		.96
VIII. Single Regiments	63	9	61	21	.300 ± .093		2.41
IX. Special Hospitals	1,088	86	4,453	538	.119 ± .022		1.53
X. Various Military Hospitals	701	63	2,864	510	.194 ± .022		1.98
XI. Army in India	73	11	1,052	423	.248 ± .050		2.67
Mean Value					.193		

* Adapted from Pearson K: Report on certain enteric fever inoculation statistics. Br Med J 2:1243–1246, 1904 (reference 9). Odds ratios added.

11). Through the rest of November to the end of December, week by week and salvo by salvo, Wright and Pearson exchanged eight more furious and sometimes insulting letters (12-19). Wright's main defense—attack might better describe it—was in essence that field trials, especially in wartime, were bound to produce inconsistency. He stressed two sources of unreliability: (1) histories of inoculation were unreliable, and (2) the clinical diagnosis of typhoid fever was even more so. The autopsy diagnosis, by contrast, was accurate, and in the peacetime Army in India, where autopsies were a requirement, (Wright said) mortality rates showed a powerful and consistent advantage of threefold or more in favor of inoculation.

After being sharply chided by Pearson for nowhere taking account of chance deviations, Wright summed up as follows (18):

Please let me remark, in passing, that it is a difference of opinion with regard to this question which is at bottom responsible for the engendering of the present discussion.

Professor Pearson, I take it, sees in the operation of chance the most important of all sources of fallacy. He demands, if I understand him right, that the effect of this factor shall be in each case set out in the form of a mathematical expression.

The weight of medical opinion is, I believe, with me when I contend against Professor Pearson that the operation of the factor of chance is not by any means the most serious cause of fallacy in medical statistics. If it were, all that would be necessary to the attainment of perfect statistics would be to insist in each case on the bringing together of considerable figures. I am confident that medical statistics are vitiated much more seriously by those other sources of fallacy which I have dealt with in my critical commentary. I refer to the fallacy of a want of conformity between the "test cases" and the "control cases", to the fallacy which is associated with the uncertainty of clinical diagnosis, and to the fallacies which are introduced by the carelessness, untrustworthiness, or ignorance of individual observers.

Issues are settled, not by statistics, but by political decision. Lord Haldane, Secretary of War, became convinced that inoculation was useful and necessary. Haldane

6   MERVYN SUSSER

got Wright a knighthood to shore his reputation as a scientist† and the Army proceeded with use of the vaccine (7).

Pearson's doubts were not ignored entirely. In a program directed by Wright's
former co-worker, Leishman, vaccine use
was monitored over a three-year period by
trained medical officers assigned to every
unit going abroad during this time (20, 21).
Exhibit 4 shows the results of this experience published by Leishman. They were
eloquent, as Leishman wrote, but less conclusive than he thought (22). The inoculated were volunteers; the diagnostic criteria were not definitive and the medical
officers who made the diagnoses in affected
cases were not necessarily blind to inoculation status; and the composition of the exposed population was not stable because
men were posted to and from units. Further, any attempt to measure duration of
exposure was confounded because some
men volunteered for vaccination after
posting abroad, sometimes in the face of a
threatened epidemic or after it, and these
records were not collected (22). The Army
Report (21) assigned men to inoculated
and uninoculated groups according to their
status at the end of the observation period,
thus inflating the duration of exposure for
the inoculated (some of whom were uninoculated for part of the time) and artefac-
tually lessening their apparent risk of contracting the disease over a given period.

Greenwood and Yule (23) corrected for
this error by reversing this procedure, a
stringent test; they assigned men to inoculated and uninoculated groups according
to their status at the beginning of the ob-

servation period, thus deflating duration
of exposure for the inoculated and artefac-
tually raising their apparent risk. This
calculation halved the relative risk of the
uninoculated compared with the inoculated from six- to three-fold, still a significant effect. By the time of World War I,
these further data had much strengthened
the case for the vaccine, and inoculation
was in regular use in the British and
French armies. The vaccine probably
saved many lives.

As Cockburn pointed out on the countervailing side, however, there is no way of
quantitatively assigning the reason for the
reduced incidence among vaccination and
the concurrent changes in clean water supplies and personal and food hygiene (22).
One should note how large the possible
costs of wrongly introducing such a vaccine could have been. A half century
passed before anyone had the courage
again to conduct a controlled prophylactic
trial of typhoid vaccine. In the 1950's such
a trial became possible because of the discovery of an antibiotic (chloromycetin) effective against typhoid fever; happily the
vaccine proved efficacious (24).

The angels were on Wright's side. We
might with profit ask ourselves why so
great a statistician as Pearson did not perceive them hovering about the head of the
man come to judgment. He rendered a sensible initial opinion. The pugnacity of the
polemics and a self-serving element in
some of Wright's arguments forced Pearson into an increasingly negative stance as
the debate proceeded. The question of
judgment must be examined in terms of
reason rather than affect, however, and it
seems to me that on a number of points
Wright sustained his argument better
than did Pearson.

Pearson used two quantifiable criteria.
The results satisfied his first strictly statistical criterion; they were well beyond
the usual *bounds for chance events*. They
did not satisfy his second criterion: the
strength of the association did not meet the

---

† Colebrook (7, p.40) states: "John Freeman has
told how it came about — on going home from work in
the early hours of the morning, they found a letter
from Lord Haldane. . . . He said there was no agreement among the Army Medical authorities about
the inoculation policy, but it had got to be adopted.
To achieve that he must build up Wright as a great
man, and the first step in that process was to make
him a knight." In this role Wright can be recognized
as Sir Colenso Ridgeon, newly knighted in the opening scenes of George Bernard Shaw's play, The Doc-
tor's Dilemma.

EXHIBIT 4*

Recent Results of Antityphoid Inoculation: Statistical table showing the results of antityphoid inoculation in sixteen units of the British Army, up to June 1, 1908

Unit	Medical Officer	Station	Date of arrival	Total strength (actual)	Inoculated			Noninoculated		
					No.	Cases	Deaths	No.	Cases	Deaths
2nd Roy. Fus	Capt. A. B. Smallman	Trimulgherry	Jan., 1905	1,013	198	10	1	815	59	9
17th Lancers	Capt. E. J. Luxmore	Merrut	Oct., 1905	616	322	3	0	294	71	12
Brigade, R.A.	Capt. E. G. Lithgow	Pindi (from Transvaal)	Nov., 1905	370	60	2	0	310	7	0
14th Hussars	Lieut. C. E. Fawcett	Bangalore	Oct., 1906	647	385	1	0	261	4	1
2nd Dorsets.	Lieut. E. G. Anthonisz	Wellington	Nov., 1906	1,107	199	1	0	908	6	0
3rd Coldstream Guards	Lieut. J. H. Graham	Cairo	Oct., 1906	705	569	1	0	136	13	1
2nd Leicesters	Lieut. H. S. Sherren	Belgaum	Oct., 1906	963	346	3	1	617	17	1
1st Connaught Rangers	Lieut. A. D. O'Carrol	Dagshai (from Malta)	Mar., 1907	483	300	0	0	183	2	1
3rd Worcesters	Lieut. W. H. Forsyth	Wynberg	Dec., 1907	900	220	0	0	680	3	0
1st Dragoon Guards	Lieut. G. H. Stevenson	Umballa	Dec., 1907	592	450	0	0	142	0	0
1st Yorks	Lieut. S. deC. O'Grady	Cairo	Jan., 1908	893	470	0	0	423	0	0
1st Suffolks.	Lieut. J. B. G. Mulligan	Malta	Dec., 1907	900	400	0	0	500	0	0
3rd Roy. Rifles	Lieut. R. W. D. Leslie	Crete	Feb., 1908	879	190	0	0	689	0	0
2nd Bedfords	Lieut. C. M. Drew	Gibraltar	Sept., 1907	700	320	0	0	380	3	1
Brigade, R.A.	Lieut. A. S. Littlejohns	Pretoria	Nov., 1907	375	247	1	0	128	2	0
1st Lan. Fus.	Lieut. F. D. G Howell	Chakrata	Dec., 1907	940	796	0	0	144	0	0
Totals				12,083	5,473	21	2	6,610	187	26

Case-incidence per 1,000.

	Inoculated	Non-inoculated
1) Among the whole of the above sixteen units	3.8	28.3
2) Among the "exposed" units, i.e., in which cases of enteric fever had occurred	6.6	39.5
3) "Exposed" units, less Royal Fusiliers (the unit inoculated with the "old vaccine")	3.7	32.8

* Taken from Leishman, W. B: Statistical table of the recent results of antityphoid inoculation. J R Army Med Corps 12:163-167, 1909 (reference 20).

8   MERVYN SUSSER

preset standard he had estimated from the only two pre-existing vaccines. While strength of association is a quantitative criterion, its application requires judgment.

Much of the passion Wright and his medical supporters felt was indirectly inspired by this criterion of strength of association. The criterion, in the form of a correlation coefficient, ignores attributable risk; it does not bring into the judgment, as we have since learned to do, the scale of benefits and costs for the population. In consequence, Pearson could be, and was, accused of callousness to the life-saving and preventive potential possessed even by this relatively inefficient vaccine.

Wright showed superior intuition with regard to a third quantifiable criterion, the ability of the trial of the vaccine to detect an effect (which I shall loosely describe as *power),* and the effect of random measurement error upon it. Wright recognized, as Pearson seemed not to, that measurement error must have suppressed the strength of the positive association that was found. As a practical consequence, had Pearson recognized the effect of the greater chance of misclassifying typhoid than of misclassifying smallpox or diphtheria, he might have been prompted to relax the level of his criterion of strength of association.

Readers will not need reminding of the importance of the power of a test (25, 26). They may need reminding, however, of the bias toward skepticism in conventional procedures of inference. Analytic strategies for avoiding false negatives are few, aside from the statistical criterion of power, and aside from the analytical elaboration of data that tests internal validity and reveals conditional or suppressed or distorted associations (2). Much statistical strategy aims to avoid false positives, inferences that give credence to causality where none exists.

Human minds seem to be more credulous than skeptical, and most people need protection against being gulled. Yet undue skepticism can be as dangerous to scientific progress as credulity. Statisticians and epidemiologists are properly professional skeptics. But we must be aware of the trained incapacity to believe in positive results. As the White Queen implied to Alice, one may have to practice believing. Why, one might ask, is the conventional level above which we reject the null hypothesis and accept a positive result set at one chance in 20, and the conventional level above which we accept the null hypothesis and reject a positive result set at one chance in five? Any disparity should rest on a weighing of the gravity of the error of accepting or rejecting an hypothesis, but the costs of rejecting a positive result seem rarely to be considered (26, 27).

Wright's intuition was superior also with regard to an unquantified criterion of judgment, namely external validation of the data by *consistency on replication.* The epidemiologist does not have the opportunities for exact replication which enable the physical scientist to demonstrate consistency. His most powerful alternative to exact replication is consistency of a finding on repeated tests (28, 29). The strength of the argument rests on the fact that diverse approaches produce similar results. There were, by Pearson's grouping, 11 independent replications of the test of the vaccine, and nine of these 11 yielded statistically significant associations. Pearson combined all the tests, and based his judgment only on the single quantitative measure of the unweighted mean value of the 11 correlation coefficients.

The force of external validation by consistency on replication was emphasized by Selvin (30). He explored the principles involved in Durkheim's studies of suicide and religious affiliation, and applied a crude probability test to show the much higher degree of significance obtained than could be attributed to any one study. Long ago, J. S. Mill stated this criterion as

JUDGMENT AND CAUSAL INFERENCE   9

the "method of agreement; all the situations are different but they have one circumstance in common." Here lies the particular cogency of the 36 studies reviewed by the Surgeon General's Committee on *Smoking and Health (31)*. This is not "the mere repetition of evidence of the same kind," as R. A. Fisher described these studies (32).

Another non-quantitative criterion of judgment necessarily applied by scientists to the interpretation of data is their *coherence,* in the sense of the reasonableness of the association in biologic terms (28). Here Wright was fortunate in his intimate knowledge of his experimental results on the bactericidal properties of the vaccine *in vitro,* as well as of the field conditions of the trial (for instance, the variability of batches of vaccine, the weaknesses of data collection and so forth). On the other side, retrospectively, Pearson seems rash in his readiness to judge the data for their coherence when he had not made a close examination of their collection and processing. He seems to have exercised what amounted to a self-denying ordinance. When Wright charged that Pearson had refused an invitation to discuss the results with Wright and his fellow committee members some time before he undertook the inspection and analysis of the results, Pearson defended his position with the claim that a statistician needed time for reflection and calculations. Noting the variability in the efficacy of the vaccine, he wrote: "It is difficult to explain this on the basis of any real theory of inoculation" (9, p. 1244). In other words, incoherence detracted from Wright's results. This was perhaps a point he thought better of, because he qualified it in a footnote and suggested some alternative explanations.

Coherence is an ultimate and yet not a necessary criterion for causality. It is, of course, essential to the overall constructs within which scientific investigation proceeds. Without it, the Baconian injunction to come to a conclusion "by proper rejec-

tions and exclusions" must remain meaningless. Only then can one conclude that an explication is coherent with other known facts. But coherence supports preexisting inference and theory. Incoherence may have a parochial or incidental explanation, as, for example, variability in the manufacture and strength of batches of vaccine. Incoherence may also have a more general explanation, in which instance it will generate new theory.* As Lilienfeld has said: "the finding of a biologically implausible association may be the first lead to this extension of knowledge" (29). In the case of the typhoid vaccine, the existing theory proved sound, and the incoherence incidental and attributable, as Wright thought, to incidental conditions.

The next example reinforces the usefulness of some of the criteria applied to the first. In April 1955, amid great fanfare, the Poliomyelitis Vaccine Evaluation Center sponsored by the National Foundation for Infantile Paralysis published its "Summary Report on the Evaluation of the 1954 Poliomyelitis Vaccine Trials" (33). In December 1955, K. A. Brownlee at the University of Chicago published an invited critique of the trial (34).

The number of schoolchildren involved in the trial was 1,829,916, and the trial cost in the region of five million dollars. Two study plans were put into effect (Exhibit 5a).

An initial plan was described as the "Observed Control" trial. Second grade children whose parents agreed they could participate were to be vaccinated. The controls were to comprise the "corresponding" first and third graders. In the event, the

---

* Sartwell (28) illuminates the point with a quotation on "nonsense correlations" from D. W. Cheever's book, The Value and Fallacy of Statistics in the Observation of Disease (1861): "It could be no more ridiculous for the stranger who passed the night in the steerage of an emigrant ship to ascribe the typhus which he there contracted, to the vermin with which bodies of the sick might be infested. An adequate cause, one reasonable in itself, must correct the coincidence of simple experience."

10   MERVYN SUSSER

"corresponding" first and third grade volunteers needed for controls could not be adequately identified from the registers, and all first and third graders were used as controls. This study covered 127 areas of 33 states with a total population of 1,080,680 children in the first, second and third grades (or 59 per cent of the total in both studies).

A second plan was described as the "Placebo Control" trial. R. Korns and M. Levin in New York State, and L. Schuman in Illinois had refused to participate unless there was a placebo control. Thomas Francis then instituted the randomized controlled trial (35).[†] Children of the first, second and third grades in the remaining study areas were invited to participate; one half of volunteers received the vaccine, the other half a placebo injection. This study covered 84 areas of 11 states with a population of 748,236 children in the first, second and third grades (41 per cent of the total of both studies).

To take first the "Placebo Control" trial (see Exhibit 5b), these results showed the vaccine to be 72 per cent effective ($100 \times (1 - R_1/R_2)$) against paralytic poliomyelitis (row *d*, third column). This result, Brownlee thought, left little doubt as to the effectiveness of the vaccine, given that there was independent random sampling and that the vaccinated and controls differed only in vaccination status. He was not satisfied, however, that this assumption held. On closer examination of the data, Brownlee noted a bias (albeit a slight one) towards greater susceptibility to poliomyelitis among the controls, as judged by preinoculation antibody levels.

Turning to the "Observed Control" trial, Brownlee dismissed the data out of hand

† Morton Levin and Abraham Lilienfeld provided this version of events. Paul (35) incorrectly attributes the controlled trial to the advice Austin Bradford Hill gave Francis who, he says, was in London when invited to direct the trial. In fact, Lilienfeld says he himself was with Francis at a conference in Atlanta when Francis received a telephone call asking him to direct the trial.

with such descriptions as "worthless" and "total folly"; the 59 per cent of the total effort devoted to this part of the trial was "stupid" and "futile". In the light of the results, and in the face of the panic and publicity about the poliomyelitis scourge at the time, it surely took courage for Brownlee to write that he felt " . . . the need for an independent confirmation."

Nonetheless, the vaccine was put into use without further trial. It proved effective (although not as effective as the oral vaccine which later replaced it), and it undoubtedly saved thousands from crippling and death. In retrospect, then, events proved Brownlee's judgment to be too skeptical, even intemperate. No doubt, he was provoked by the heat of debate and publicity, for the National Foundation for Infantile Paralysis had brought large-scale publicity techniques to bear on a scientific issue for the first time, and the pressure to produce had led to risky decisions, even wrong decisions, with some unhappy consequences for the vaccinated (35–37). It was a time, too, when for many the randomized controlled trial had still to establish itself as the preferred means of testing a mode of intervention.

Brownlee, doing battle on behalf of the randomized controlled trial, seems to have blinkered himself from all other evidence. He pointed to two results that demonstrated the "futility of the work in the observed areas." First, non-participants (mainly refusals) had different rates of school absenteeism and were of lower social class than volunteers, and second, they had lower rates of poliomyelitis (as determined from the rate among those given placebo). Thus, it was obviously improper in the "Observed Control" trial, all will agree, to compare the vaccinated second grade *volunteers* with the *total population* of the first and third grades, as was done in the summary report (Row *i* in Exhibit 5b). This comparison runs the risk of confounding by social class and other factors related to poliomyelitis incidence,

JUDGMENT AND CAUSAL INFERENCE   11

EXHIBIT 5a

Study plans for poliomyelitis vaccine field trial, 1954*

"Placebo Control" Trial		"Observed Control" Trial
a. Half 1st, 2nd, 3rd grade volunteers; randomly assigned. $N = 200,745$.	*Vaccinated*	e. 2nd grade volunteers. $N = 221,998$.
b. Half 1st, 2nd, 3rd grade volunteers, randomly assigned. $N = 201,229$.	*Controls*	f. All 1st and 3rd grade children. $N = 725,173$.
c. 1st, 2nd, 3rd grade refusals. $N = 338,778$.	*Non-participants* (Refusals, absentees, etc.)	g. 2nd grade. $N = 123,605$.

* Adapted from Vaccine Evaluation Center: Evaluation of the Field Trial of Poliomyelitis Vaccine. Summary Report. Ann Arbor, MI, University of Michigan, 1955 (reference 33).

EXHIBIT 5b

Comparison of poliomyelitis among vaccinated and controls under two study plans: Rates per 100,000*

	All cases	All polio	Paralytic	Non-paralytic	Non-polio
	"Placebo Control" Trial				
a. Vaccinated: 1st, 2nd, 3rd grade	41	28	16	12	12
b. Placebo: 1st, 2nd, 3rd grades	81	71	57	13	10
c. Non-participants†: 1st, 2nd, 3rd grades	54	46	36	11	7
d. Ratio of Vaccinated to Placebo	.506	.394	.280	.923	.120
	"Observed Control" Trial				
e. Vaccinated: 2nd grade	34	25	17	8	9
f. Unvaccinated: 1st and 3rd grades	61	54	46	8	6
g. Non-participants†: 2nd grade	53	44	35	9	10
h. Total: 2nd grade	41	32	23	8	9
i. Ratio of vaccinated 2nd grade to all 1st and 3rd grades	.557	.462	.369	1.0	1
j. Ratio of all 2nd grade to all 1st and 3rd grades	.672	.592	.50	1.0	1.5

* Adapted from Vaccine Evaluation Center: Evaluation of the Field Trial of Poliomyelitis Vaccine. Summary Report. Ann Arbor, MI, University of Michigan, 1955 (reference 33).

† Mainly refusals.

in addition to the risk created by the imperfect age match across school grade.

Yet, by the criterion of consistency on replication, and by the criterion of coherence, the "Observed Control" trial provided valuable support, unrecognized by Brownlee, for the "Placebo Control" trial. Thus, we are back with the question of judgment. First, with regard to external validation by consistency on replication, note that the incidence of poliomyelitis in several categories of increasing diagnostic refinement is virtually identical in the "Placebo Control" and "Observed Control" areas both among the vaccinated and among the non-participants.

Further, in the "Observed Control" trial a legitimate comparison can be made between the *total* second grade population, vaccinated and unvaccinated, and the *total* first and third grade populations (Exhibit 5b, row *j*). The comparison can be taken as a stringent test of the total program in the field, since the closer observation of vaccinated children, solely in the second grade, was likely to bring more poliomyelitis cases to light in the second grade than in the first and third grade controls.* The vaccine remains effective, although less so (50 per cent), by this test ($\chi^2 = 29.14$; d.f. $= 1$; $p < .001$).

This comparison, in the double-barrelled design of "placebo" and "observed" controls, would also have proved a safeguard against a contingency that did not, but might have occurred. It is not inconceivable that in the "Placebo Control" trial a fully effective vaccine could have produced a level of herd immunity in the population that would have protected the placebo controls to a degree that significant differences between them and the vaccinated did not clearly emerge. Contamination of the control group was a lesser likelihood in the "Observed Control" design, since first and third grade controls were less likely to commingle with the vaccinated second graders, whereas in the "Placebo Control" design the vaccinated and the controls were in the same classroom.

With regard to the criterion of coherence, the most refined diagnosis, and hence the most precise results, were to be expected among paralytic cases, and in both studies it is these cases which contribute the great part of the positive result. Further, as noted above, lower socioeconomic classes had a known lower incidence of poliomyelitis and a demonstrated lower level of participation in the study. For this reason, the dilution of the result seen in the "Observed Control" trial was coherent and to be anticipated, since the control incidence rates were lowered by the inclusion of non-participants among them (not by intention, it seems, but because of flawed execution of the registration of acceptance and refusal among controls in the first and third grades).

Nonetheless, the existence of the "Observed Control" provided a coherent rebut-

tal against one critical interpretation of the results of the "Placebo Control" design. The higher incidence of poliomyelitis among the placebo controls than among the vaccinated, it was argued by the critics, could be the result, not of the protection of the vaccinated, but of provocation by inoculation, just as previously poliomyelitis had been found to be provoked by other inoculations. Francis (38) was able to refute the suggestion from the data (unpublished) on volunteers who received no injections in the "Observed Control" areas. The estimated risk in the "Observed Control" areas for volunteers who received no injections (as compared with those who refused participation) was the same as the risk in the "Placebo Control" areas of those who received placebo injections (as compared with those who refused participation).

Brownlee took the position that the difference between the evidence from a blind randomized prophylactic trial and any other is absolute. He cited the Summary Report: "In observed areas where only those second grade children whose parents requested participation were vaccinated, the problem of establishing the control population was more complex", and he commented: "It is perfectly true to say that it is more complex, but to indulge in understatements of this order of magnitude is to be misleading. The plain fact is that it is impossible." Brownlee was misled by Fisher's central dogma of the randomized trial. Differences in strength of inference from experimental and observational studies are relative, not absolute, as anyone who has conducted large experimental field trials will know, and to test their validity requires that we bring to bear all possible criteria of judgment to all the data.

The next example bears on the controversy about the effects of smoking. Judgment failed two major statisticians, one of whom many class among the greatest of all. Joseph Berkson and R. A. Fisher both

---

* Although the Summary Report (33) makes little of this comparison, Alexander Langmuir tells me that he and William Cochran insisted that the essential data be included in the report.

disputed the causal associations of smoking with lung cancer. Berkson (39, 40) advanced a multitude of arguments, some good and most less good—like Pearson, at one point he proposed the mere unreliability of data (smoking histories and death certificates) as a reason for the finding of a spurious positive association and, at another point, the apparent incoherence of some of the results—but he devoted his major attack to the judgmental criterion of specificity. Here Berkson took his stand on ground prepared for him by Yerushalmy and Palmer (41) who argued that "specificity of effect" was one essential of Koch's postulates. In chronic disease too, he held, specificity should be sought. A characteristic is specific to a disease "when . . . similar relationships do not exist with a variety of characteristics and with many disease entities when such relationships are not predictable on physiologic, pathologic, experimental or epidemiologic grounds. In general, the lower the frequency of these other associations, the higher is the specificity of the observed association and the higher the validity of the causal inference" (41, pp. 38–39).

By the term *specificity of association*, then, we describe the precision with which the occurrence of one variable will predict the occurrence of another. The ideal, a one-to-one relationship, encompasses the element of strength of association as well as of precision, and might be better reduced to the statement that one thing, and only one thing, causes one effect and only one effect. Departures from the ideal occur first where many things are posed as causes of a single effect, and second where a single thing is posed as the cause of many effects. In the smoking controversy, Berkson was perturbed by the second type of departure from the ideal in the smoking data, i.e., where one thing has many effects. He noted the congeries of manifestations found in association with smoking, and he argued that such non-specificity casts doubt on any causal relationship. He

carried the attack forward by analogy. He pointed to the extraordinarily regular association of marital status—in the order of married, single, divorced—with overall mortality from many specific diseases. He offered, as more likely than some of the causal associations considered by others, such explanations as systematic bias in registered data. The equally non-specific associations of smoking with disease, Berkson held, led to equally infirm inferences of causality.

Arguments that demand specificity are fallacious, if not absurd. There can be no logical reason why any identifiable factor, and especially an unrefined one, should not have multiple effects (2, 28, 29, 42). To take Berkson's own analogy, marital status, in the form of transition into widowhood, has since been shown to be a highly probable cause of suicides, of entry into psychiatric care, and of cirrhosis of the liver (43–48). Other associations will not prove causal, but there is surely more to come. By now it is evident that the associations of health disorders with smoking depend on a variety of mechanisms, some causal and some not. Specificity enhances the plausibility of causal inference, but lack of specificity does not negate it.

Fisher's major attack on the smoking and lung cancer hypothesis was around the judgmental criterion of the *time-order and logical structure* of causal and outcome variables (although he too attacked on grounds of incoherence) (32). Predisposition poses a major problem in inferring the time-order of variables. As a latent manifestation of an outcome variable, predisposition must cast doubt on the precedence in time of supposedly independent causal variables. Fisher suggested that smokers could be self-selected from among persons with a genetic predisposition both to smoking and to lung cancer, and pointed for supporting evidence to the association between genetic constitution and smoking habits.

These associations between personality

14   MERVYN SUSSER

type and smoking habit pose the same difficulties for inferring time-order among
variables as all others measured at the
same point in time. While predisposition
cannot be excluded, its presence has certainly not been demonstrated. Vital links
in the logical structure of this counter-
hypothesis are missing. The relevant personality traits have even now not been
linked with lung cancer, let alone been
shown to antedate the disease. If this link
with the disease were to be supplied, the
association of the rising trend in the frequency of lung cancer with smoking and
its distribution among the sexes, and,
most of all, the overwhelming strength of
the association (49, 50), would require at
the least that smoking be a crucial intervening variable between the predisposition to lung cancer and its manifestations.
(There are several other criteria of judgment by which this argument can be pursued, as has been ably done by authors
beginning in the early days of the controversy (31, 49)).

Fisher chose a criterion for attack on
which many inferences of causality are
vulnerable; in observational studies the
criterion of time-order is perhaps the most
difficult to defend. In order finally to determine time-order and logical structure
among variables, our main reliance must
be on design: we use incidence rather than
prevalence measures, cohort rather than
case-control studies. Here, cohort studies
and the effects of stopping smoking on
mortality have settled the question for
most of us (51). Recent attacks on the
smoking hypothesis add nothing essentially new to the arguments of Fisher and
Berkson.

In conclusion, this paper should not be
construed as an attack on statistical inference or on major statisticians, but as a
demonstration of the fallibility of judgment even among those with superb technical equipment, and of the need for developing the means of decision-making. Some
injunctions may perhaps be drawn from

the review of these few case histories. One
should be aware of bias toward negative
judgments, which require as much caution
as positive judgments, recognize that the
difference between types of evidence is relative and not absolute, and apply all available criteria of judgment to any particular
instance. Perhaps we may advance beyond
our present limitations by systematizing
our criteria of judgment, and by expanding
the number and type of available criteria.

REFERENCES

1. Raiffa H: Decision Analysis: Introductory Lec-
   tures on Choices under Uncertainty. New York,
   Addison Wesley, 1970
2. Susser M: Causal Thinking in the Health Sciences: Concepts and Strategies of Epidemiology.
   New York, Oxford University Press, 1973
3. Susser M, Adelstein AM (eds.): Introduction to
   Vital Statistics: A Memorial Volume of Selections from the Reports and Writings of William
   Farr. Edited by NA Humphreys. London, Sanitary Institute of Great Britain, 1885. Reprinted
   for the New York Academy of Medicine. Me-
   tuchen, NJ, Scarecrow Press, Inc., 1975
4. Humphreys NA (ed.): Vital Statistics: A Memorial Volume of Selections from the Reports and
   Writings of William Farr. London, Sanitary Institute of Great Britain, 1885
5. Serfling RE: Historical review of epidemic theory. Hum Biol 24:145–166, 1952
6. Brownlee J: Historical note on Farr's theory of
   the epidemic. Br Med J 2:250–252, 1915
7. Colebrook L: Almroth Wright: Provocative Doc-
   tor and Thinker. London, Heinemann, 1954
8. Wright AE: A Short Treatise on Anti-typhoid
   Inoculation. Westminster, Archibald Constable
   & Co, London, 1904
9. Pearson K: Report on certain enteric fever inoculation statistics. Br Med J 2:1243–1246, 1904
10. Wright AE: Antityphoid inoculation. Br Med J
    2:1233, 1904
11. Editorial. Br Med J 2:1259–1261, 1904
12. Wright AE: Antityphoid inoculation. Br Med J
    2:1343–1345, 1904
13. Pearson K: Antityphoid inoculation. Br Med J
    2:1432, 1904
14. Wright AE: Antityphoid inoculation. Br Med J
    2:1489–1491, 1904
15. Pearson K: Antityphoid inoculation. Br Med J
    2:1542, 1904
16. Wright AE: Antityphoid inoculation. Br Med J
    2:1614, 1904
17. Pearson K: Antityphoid inoculation. Br Med J
    2:1667–1668, 1904
18. Wright AE: Antityphoid inoculation. Br Med J
    2:1727, 1904
19. Pearson K: Antityphoid inoculation. Br Med J
    2:1775–1776, 1904
20. Leishman WB: Statistical table of the recent

results of antityphoid inoculation. J R Army Med Corps 12:163–167, 1909

21. Report of Antityphoid Committee, G. B. (1912). London, Her Majesty's Stationery Office, 1913

22. Cockburn WC: The early history of typhoid vaccination. J R Army Med Corps 101:171–185, 1955

23. Greenwood M, Yule GU: Statistics of antityphoid and anticholera inoculation and interpretation of such statistics in general epidemiology. Proc R Soc Med 8:113–194, 1915

24. Cvjetanovic BB: Field trials of typhoid vaccines. Am J Public Health 47:578–581, 1957

25. Neyman J, Pearson ES: On the use and interpretation of certain test criteria of statistical inference. Biometrika 20:175–240, 264–299, 1928

26. Neyman J, Pearson ES: On the problem of the most efficient of statistical hypotheses. Philos Trans R Soc Lond 231A:289–337, 1933

27. Lehmann EL: Some principles of the theory of testing hypotheses. Ann Math Stat 21:1–26, 1950

28. Sartwell PE: "On the methodology of investigations of etiologic factors in chronic diseases": Further comments. J Chron Dis 11:61–63, 1960

29. Lilienfeld AM: "On the methodology of investigations of etiologic factors in chronic diseases": Some comments. J Chronic Dis 10:41–46, 1959

30. Selvin HC: Durkheim's suicide and problems of empirical research. Am J Sociol 63:607–619, 1958

31. United States Dept. of Health, Education and Welfare: Smoking and Health: Report of the Advisory Committee to the Surgeon General. Washington DC, USGPO, 1964

32. Fisher RA: Smoking and the Cancer Controversy. Edinburgh, Oliver and Boyd, 1959, p 11

33. Vaccine Evaluation Center: Evaluation of the Field Trial of Poliomyelitis Vaccine. Summary Report. Ann Arbor, MI, University of Michigan, 1955

34. Brownlee KA: Statistics of the 1954 polio vaccine trials. J Am Stat Ass 50:1005–1013, 1955

35. Paul JR: A History of Poliomyelitis. New Haven, CN, Yale University Press, 1971

36. Meier P: Safety testing of poliomyelitis vaccine. Science 125:1067–1071, 1957

37. Langmuir A: The surveillance of communicable diseases of national importance. N Engl J Med 268:182–192, 1963

38. Francis T: Symposium on controlled vaccine field trials: Poliomyelitis. Am J Public Health 47:283–287, 1957

39. Berkson J: Smoking and cancer of the lung. Proc Staff Meeting of the Mayo Clinic 35:367–385, 1960

40. Berkson J: Mortality and marital status. Am J Public Health 52:1318–1329, 1962

41. Yerushalmy J, Palmer CE: On the methodology of investigations of etiologic factors in chronic diseases. J Chronic Dis 10:27–40, 1959

42. MacMahon B, Pugh TF, Ipsen J: Epidemiologic Methods. Boston, Little, Brown, 1960

43. Ciocco A: On the mortality in husbands and wives. Hum Biol 12:508–531, 1940

44. Ciocco A: On the mortality in brother-sister and husband-wife pairings. Hum Biol 13:189–202, 1941

45. Kraus AS, Lilienfeld AM: Some epidemiologic aspects of the high mortality rate in the young widowed group. J Chronic Dis 10:207–217, 1959

46. MacMahon B, Pugh TF: Suicide in the widowed. Am J Epidemiol 81:23–31, 1965

47. Stein ZA, Susser MW: Widowhood and mental illness. Br J Prev Soc Med 23:106–110, 1969

48. McNeil D, Kelsey JL: Cirrhosis mortality among widows. Paper presented at the Seventh International Meeting of the International Epidemiological Association, University of Sussex, England, August 17–21, 1974

49. Cornfield J, Haenszel W, Hammond EC, et al: Smoking and lung cancer: Recent evidence and a discussion of some questions. J Natl Cancer Inst 22:173–203, 1959

50. Bross IDJ: Pertinency of an extraneous variable. J Chronic Dis 20:487–495, 1967

51. Doll R: The age distribution of cancer: Implications for models of carcinogenesis. J R Stat Soc 134:133–166, 1971

Part II

Developments in Theory and Quantitative Methods

Part II is meant to serve as a source of articles that introduced, to epidemiologists at least, ideas and quantitative methods that have become central to epidemiologic theory and practice. In some cases, most notably Sheehe [1962], the article was profoundly original but largely ignored, and is included here to exhibit the earliest work on the topic. In other cases, such as Miettinen [1976], the central concepts had for the most part been anticipated in the literature, but the article was the first to explicate and synthesize them in a fashion leading to widespread dissemination and understanding.

None of the articles, except Sheehe's, requires any mathematics beyond high school algebra for full appreciation. I encourage readers without much mathematical knowledge not to be intimidated by the mathematical arguments they will encounter here; the text of each article has much to offer. In any case it would be better to skip over bits of algebra than to skip the whole article (although for full appreciation one should work through the algebra as well).

I have purposely excluded articles on misclassification and matching, primarily because of lack of space, and also because literature in both areas tended to be either unclear or heavily mathematical until the late 1970's.

II–1.

Joseph Berkson: Limitations of the Application of Fourfold Table Analysis to Hospital Data. Biometrics 1946; 2:47–53.

Berkson's 1946 article, "Limitations of the Application of Fourfold Table Analysis to Hospital Data," is the earliest algebraic analysis of an epidemiologic selection bias of which I am aware. In one sense Berkson was far ahead of his time: though his article became famous within the field during the three decades covered by this collection, over the same period I could find no algebraic analyses of other selection bias phenomena (although reviews of Berkson's arguments were common).

Described in modern terminology, Berkson studied the phenomenon that diseases can appear associated in a hospital-based case-control study solely on account of higher admission rates among persons with multiple conditions, even if the conditions affect admission rates independently. This phenomenon came to be known as "Berkson's bias," a term rumored to have been deplored by Berkson since it suggested that Berkson committed the bias, rather than discovered it.

An unfortunate aspect of the history of Berkson's paper has been a tendency to overlook the fact that the phenomenon described by Berkson was *not* a general problem of case-control studies. Kraus [1954] was perhaps the earliest author to indicate the limitations of Berkson's argument. For Berkson's bias to occur, it was necessary that both the outcome under study *and* the putative risk factor independently affect hospitalization rates. Kraus pointed out that typical study factors are not active diseases, and therefore are unlikely to affect hospitalization rates; thus Berkson's bias would not be a threat in most studies.

Although the practical importance of the specific phenomenon studied by Berkson remains debatable, some empirical evidence for its occurrence has been offered [Roberts et al., 1978], and there can be little doubt that Berkson's contribution helped stimulate many of the more recent analyses of selection and response biases.

References:
Kraus AS. The use of hospital data in studying the association between a characteristic and a disease. Pub Health Rep 1954; 69:1211–1214.

Roberts RS, Spitzer WO, Delmore T, Sackett DL. An empirical demonstration of Berkson's bias. J Chron Dis 1978; 31:119–128.

LIMITATIONS OF THE APPLICATION OF
FOURFOLD TABLE ANALYSIS TO HOSPITAL DATA*

JOSEPH BERKSON, M.D.,

Division of Biometry and Medical Statistics, Mayo Clinic,
Rochester, Minnesota

In the biologic laboratory we have a method of procedure for determining the effect of an agent or process that may be considered typical. It consists in dividing a group of animals into two cohorts, one considered the "experimental group," the other the "control." On the experimental group some variable is brought to play; the control is left alone. The results are set up as in table 1-a. If the results show that the ratio $a:a+b$ is different from the ratio $c:c+d$, it is considered demonstrated that the process brought to bear on the experimental group has had a significant effect.

A similar method is prevalent in statistical practice, which I venture to think has come into authority because of its apparent equivalence to the experimental procedure. In Biometrika it is referred to as the fourfold table and it is used as a paradigm of statistical analysis. The usual arrangement is that given in table 1-b. The entries, a, b, c and d are manipulated arithmetically to determine whether there is any correlation between A and B. A considerable number of indices have been elaborated to measure this correlation. Pearson has given the formula for calculating the product-moment correlation coefficient from a fourfold table on the assumption that the distribution of both variates is normal; Yule has an index of association for the fourfold table; there are the chi-square test and others. In essence, however, all these indices measure in different ways whether and how much, in comparison with the variation of random sampling, the ratio $a:a+b$ differs from the ratio $c:c+d$. If the difference departs significantly from zero, there is said to be correlation, and the correlation is *the* greater the greater the difference.

Now there is a distinction between the method as used in the laboratory and as

*This paper was presented in somewhat different form at a meeting of the American Statistical Association in 1938. Recent inquiries have prompted its publication at this time.

47

applied in practical statistics. In the experimental situation, the groups, *B* and not *B*, are selected *before* the subgroupings, *A* and not *A*, are effected; that is, we start with a total group of unaffected animals. In the statistical application, the groupings, *B* and not *B*, are made *after* the subgroupings, *A* and not *A*, are already determined; that is, all the effects are already produced *before* the investigation starts. In the end, the tables of the results which are drawn up *look* alike for the two cases, but they have been arrived at differently. Correlative to this difference, a different interpretation may apply to the results, and this paper deals with a specific case of a kind that arises frequently in a medical clinic or a hospital. I take an example.

There was prevalent an impression that cholecystic disease is a provocative agent in the causation or aggravation of diabetes. In certain medical circles, the gall bladder was being removed as a treatment for diabetes. The authorities of a hospital wish to know whether their accumulated records of incidence, examined statistically, support this practice. On the face of it, it would appear that we have here the typical and elementary problem of the comparision of rates in a fourfold table. The total population of patients for a period is to be divided into two groups, "diabetes" and "no diabetes" and the rate of incidence of cholecystitis in the one compared with the rate in the other. Accordingly, table 2 was set up.

Table 2 shows a significant difference indicating positive correlation between cholecystitis and diabetes. An objection which might be brought against this particular tabulation is that the "not diabetes" group consisting as it does of all patients without diabetes, will contain a variety of diagnoses, some of which may themselves be correlated with cholecystitis, even as diabetes may be; hence the control may be considered not good. To meet this objection we do not select for the control group the entire nondiabetic population, but take a diagnosis which cannot reasonably be thought to be correlated with cholecystitis and use this as a criterion for the control group. I took, in fact, several refractive errors of the sort for which patients

come to the clinic for glasses as such a diagnostic group, and table 3 was the result.

Again we see that the difference is positive and significant in comparison with the probable error, and the usual judgment would be that cholecystitis and diabetes are positively correlated. Of course, in any detailed analysis we should wish to keep age and sex constant, inquire into the reliability of the diagnoses, and so forth. But the point referred to in this paper has no relation to such questions, and for the sake of the argument we shall consider that all such factors have been adequately controlled. Even so, do the results permit any conclusion as to whether cholecystitis is biologically correlated with diabetes?

Since the hospital population comes from the general population, let us begin there. For the sake of simplification, we shall consider only the three diseases referred to, cholecystitis, diabetes and refractive errors. If the incidence of these conditions in the general population is represented by p_c, p_d and p_r and there is no correlation between the diseases, we have for the constitution of the population the expressions shown in table 4, in which n_d is the number having diabetes but not having cholecystitis nor refractive errors, n_{dc} those having diabetes and cholecystitis but not having refractive errors, n_{dcr} those having diabetes, cholecystitis and refractive errors, n_o those having none of these diseases, and so forth. N is the total population. If we assume for illustrative purposes, a population of 10,000,000 persons, and $p_d = 0.01$, $p_c = 0.03$, and $p_r = 0.10$, the numbers of the various constituents are given in table 4. From these figures we may set up two fourfold tables as before (table 5).

In both parts of table 5 it is seen that the difference of the pertinent ratios is zero, which is as it should be, since there is no correlation. This result, of course, could have been foreseen without this computation but I desired to establish the numbers for use later. Now suppose we follow that portion of the population which gets to the hospital. For this purpose we must develop some elementary relationships.

We shall suppose that associated with each

particular disease is a definite probability that its victims will be selected for the hospital. That is, we shall suppose that a person who has cholecystitis has a certain definite probability of being drawn to the hospital because of the presence of that disease alone, and so for other diseases. Furthermore, for simplicity we shall say that these selective probabilities operate independently, as though a person who had two diseases were like Siamese twins, each one of whom had one disease, so that the probability of the twins' coming to the hospital is the probability of either one getting there, but the presence of one disease does not affect the other in any way. Let the selective rates be represented by s_1, s_2, s_3, and so forth and their complements $(1 - s)$ be represented by t_1, t_2, t_3, and so forth, the number in the general population by n and the number in the hospital by n'. Then, we have the following equations:

$$n'_1 = n_1(1-t_1) = n_1(s_1)$$
$$n'_{12} = n_{12}(1-t_1 t_2) = n_{12}(s_1+s_2-s_1 s_2)$$
$$n'_{123} = n_{123}(1-t_1t_2t_3) = n_{123}(s_1+s_2+s_3-s_1s_2-s_1s_3-s_2s_3+s_1s_2s_3)$$

From these relationships an interesting conclusion can at once be drawn. Suppose all the s's are equal, but small; then the following ratios will result:

$$\frac{n'_{12}}{n'_1} = \frac{n_{12}}{n_1}(2-s) = \text{approximately, } \frac{n_{12}}{n_1} \times 2$$

$$\frac{n'_{123}}{n'_1} = \frac{n_{123}}{n_1}(3-3s+s^2) = \text{approximately, } \frac{n_{123}}{n_1} \times 3$$

From these equations it is seen that the ratio of multiple diagnoses to single diagnoses in the hospital will always be greater than in the general population; for two diagnoses the ratio will be about twice that of the general population, for three diagnoses about three times, and so forth.

Let us now apply the appropriate factors of selection to the various constituents of the hypothetical general population which have been enumerated. Assuming as a simple instance that all the selective probabilities are equal and have the value 0.05, the frequencies given in tables 6 and 7 will result.

We see here that though in the general population, the incidence of cholecystitis was identical among the persons who had diabetes and the persons who had refractive errors, in the hospital population the incidence was less in the diabetic group than in the control group, giving an appearance of a small negative correlation, and this in the face of the fact that we have assumed equality of selective rates for the various diseases.

In general the selective rates can be assumed to be anything but equal for different diseases. Various circumstances, such as the severity of the symptoms, the amenability of the disease to treatment by a local physician or the reputation of a particular hospital for treatment of particular diseases, will determine the probability that a specific disease will bring its victim to a particular hospital. To see the effect of a variation in selective rates, let us hypothesize some values which will differ among themselves as follows: $s_c = 0.15$, $s_d = 0.05$, $s_r = 0.20$. The resulting numbers of the various constituents of the population that will come into the hospital are shown in table 8 and the fourfold table drawn up from these figures is given as table 9.

We now find that the incidence of cholecystitis in the diabetic group is about twice that of the control. This would show, so far as the hospital population is concerned, a positive correlation between cholecystitis and diabetes, but it would be quite unrepresentative of the situation in the general population and of no biologic significance.

The relationships dealt with arithmetically in the previous tables are given algebraically as follows:

$$p'_{1.2} = \frac{p_1q_3(1-t_1t_2)+p_1p_3(1-t_1t_2t_3)}{p_1q_3(1-t_1t_2)+q_1q_3(1-t_2)+p_1p_3(1-t_1t_2t_3)+p_3q_1(1-t_2t_3)}$$

$$p'_{1.3} = \frac{p_1(1-t_1t_3)}{p_1(1-t_1t_3)+q_1(1-t_3)}$$

49

Where

$p'_{1.2}$ is the incidence in the hospital population of condition 1 among persons who have condition 2

$p'_{1.3}$ is the incidence in the hospital population of condition 1 in the control group who have condition 3

p_1, p_2, and p_3 are the independent probabilities in the general population of conditions 1, 2 and 3, $q = 1 - p$

t_1, t_2, and t_3 are the complements $(1-s)$ of the independent selective probabilities s_1, s_2 and s_3 applying to condition 1, 2 and 3

Comment

The assumption made in the text that a probability can be assigned to every disease, which gives the chance that a patient suffering from that disease alone, will come to the hospital is, I think, in general accord with the actual mechanism by which such a patient is selected for the hospital population. The assumption that these probabilities operated independently in an individual who is suffering from more than one disease is doubtless oversimple. In general we may guess that if a patient is suffering from two diseases, each disease is itself aggravated in its symptoms and more likely to be noted by the patient. So far as this difference of fact from assumption goes, its effect would be to increase relatively the representation of multiple diagnoses in the hospital, and in general to increase the discrepancy between hospital and parent population, even more than if the probabilities were independent.

It appears from the development that it is hazardous to apply in a hospital population the method of the fourfold table analysis for an inquiry into the correlation of diseases. This applies also to other similar problems, as for instance whether the incidence of say, heart disease, is different for laborers and farmers, if it is known that laborers and farmers are not represented in the hospital in the proportion that they occur in the community. However, the formulas given indicate some special cases in which comparison is not basically invalid. If the selective rate for any particular condition is zero, the relative incidence of that condition in several disease groups may be validly examined, regardless of the selective rates affecting the other groups. This refers to inquiries in which for instance eye color or anthropologic type is examined in various disease groups to ascertain whether there is correlation between these characters and disease. If each of the disease groups examined consists of only one disease, for example, diabetes or refractive errors but not both, and if the selective rates for these two groups do not differ appreciably then also it is valid to compare the incidence in them of cholecystitis, even though the latter disease is not fairly represented in the hospital.

Except for such cases there does not appear to be any ready way of correcting the spurious correlation existing in the hospital population by any device that does not involve the acquisition of data which would themselves answer the primary question. For instance the device sometimes used of setting up in the hospital sample a one-to-one control so that both groups examined have the same number of cases and are identical as regards say, age and sex does not touch the difficulties referred

Table 1
Fourfold Tables

a				b			
Typical of experimental situation				Statistical form			
Group	Effect	No effect	Total	Group	A	Not A	Total
Experimental	a	b	a+b	B	a	b	a+b
Control	c	d	c+d	Not B	c	d	c+d
Total	a+c	b+d	a+b+c+d	Total	a+c	b+d	a+b+c+d

to here. It is to be emphasized that the spurious correlations referred to are not a consequence of any assumptions regarding biologic forces, or the direct selection of correlated probabilities, but are the result merely of the ordinary compounding of independent probabilities. The same results as shown here would appear if the sampling were applied to randomly distributed cards instead of patients.

Table 2

Relation of cholecystitis to diabetes—hospital population

	A Cholecystitis	Not A Not cholecystitis	Total
B: Diabetes	28	548	576
Not B: Not diabetes	1,326	39,036	40,362
Total	1,354	39,584	40,938
Cholecystitis in diabetic group			4.86%
Cholecystitis in control group (not diabetic)			3.28%
Difference			+1.58%±0.5%

Table 3

Relation of cholecystitis to diabetes—hospital population, refractive errors used as control

	A Cholecystitis	Not A Not cholecystitis	Total
Diabetes	28	548	576
Refractive errors	68	2,606	2,674
Total	96	3,154	3,250
Cholecystitis in diabetic group			4.86%
Cholecystitis in control group (refractive errors)			2.54%
Difference			+2.32%±0.5%

Table 4

Constitution of general population, various diseases

$$n_d = p_d q_e q_r \times N = 87,300$$
$$n_e = p_e q_d q_r \times N = 267,300$$
$$n_r = p_r q_d q_e \times N = 960,300$$
$$n_{de} = p_d p_e q_r \times N = 2,700$$
$$n_{dr} = p_d p_r q_e \times N = 9,700$$
$$n_{er} = p_e p_r q_d \times N = 29,700$$
$$n_{der} = p_d p_e p_r \times N = 300$$
$$n_0 = q_d q_e q_r \times N = 8,642,700$$

$$N = 10,000,000$$
$$p_d = 0.01, \quad p_e = 0.03, \quad p_r = 0.10$$
$$q_d = 0.99, \quad q_e = 0.97, \quad q_r = 0.90$$

Table 5
Cholecystitis and diabetes, general population

	Cholecystitis	Not cholecystitis	Total		Cholecystitis	Not cholecystitis	Total
Diabetes	3,000	97,000	100,000	Diabetes	3,000	97,00J	100,000
Not diabetes	297,000	9,603,000	9,900,000	Refractive errors	29,700	960,300	990,000
Total	300,000	9,700,000	10,000,000	Total	32,700	1,057,300	1,090,000

Cholecystitis in diabetic group	3%	Cholecystitis in diabetic group	3%
Cholecystitis in control group (nondiabetic)	3%	Cholecystitis in control group (refractive errors)	3%
Difference	0%	Difference	0%

Table 6
Enumeration of hospital population for $s_d = s_c = s_r = 0.05$

General population numbers	f*	Hospital population, expected numbers
n_d = 87,300	0.05	n'_d = 4,365
n_c = 267,300	0.05	n'_c = 13,365
n_r = 960,300	0.05	n'_r = 48,015
n_{dc} = 2,700	0.0975	n'_{dc} = 263
n_{dr} = 9,700	0.0975	n'_{dr} = 946
n_{cr} = 29,700	0.0975	n'_{cr} = 2,896
n_{dcr} = 300	0.142625	n'_{dcr} = 43
n_o = 8,642,700	0	n'_o = 0

*The fraction of the specified individuals which is selected for the hospital under the operation of the selective forces s. It is equal to 1 minus the products of the appropriate t's; for example $f_{dcr} = 1 - t_d t_c t_r$.

Table 7
*Cholecystitis and diabetes, hospital population:
expected numbers for $s_c = s_d = s_r = 0.05$*

	Cholecystitis	Not cholecystitis	Total
Diabetes	306	5,311	5,617
Refractive errors	2,896	48,015	50,911
Total	3,202	53,326	56,528

Cholecystitis in diabetic group	5.45%
Cholecystitis in control group (refractive errors)	5.69%
Difference	−0.24%

Table 8
Enumeration of a hospital population for
$s_c=0.15$, $s_d=0.05$, $s_r=0.20$

General population numbers	f	Hospital population, expected numbers
n_d = 87,300	0.05	n'_d = 4,365
n_c = 267,300	0.15	n'_c = 40,095
n_r = 960,300	0.20	n'_r = 192,060
n_{dc} = 2,700	0.1925	n'_{dc} = 520
n_{dr} = 9,700	0.24	n'_{dr} = 2,328
n_{cr} = 29,700	0.32	n'_{cr} = 9,504
n_{dcr} = 300	0.354	n'_{dcr} = 106
n_0 = 8,642,700	0	n'_0 = 0

Table 9

Cholecystitis and diabetes, hospital population
expected numbers for $s_c=0.15$, $s_d=0.05$, $s_r=0.20$

	Cholecystitis	Not cholecystitis	Total
Diabetes	626	6,693	7,319
Refractive errors	9,504	192,060	201,564
Total	10,130	198,753	208,883
Cholecystitis in diabetic group			8.55%
Cholecystitis in control group (refractive errors)			4.72%
Difference			+3.83%

II–2.

Jerome Cornfield: A Method of Estimating Comparative Rates from Clinical Data. Applications to Cancer of the Lung, Breast, and Cervix. Journal of the National Cancer Institute 1951; 11:1269–1275.

Cornfield's "A Method of Estimating Comparative Rates from Clinical Data" is perhaps the most famous paper in this collection, for, as every beginning epidemiology student should know, it introduced the use of the odds ratio as an estimate of relative risk from case-control studies. It is interesting, though, that this procedure was not the only or even the first method introduced in the paper. Cornfield fully appreciated the importance of looking at absolute as well as relative risks, and before introducing the odds ratio formula Cornfield gave a method of estimating absolute rates from case-control data using an external estimate of the total (crude) rate in the source population (this method is algebraically equivalent to Bayes' theorem).

A few aspects of the paper seem dated, most notably Cornfield's failure (in my view) to distinguish properly between period prevalence and incidence rates. Types of incidence were not distinguished in Cornfield's era [Vandenbroucke, 1985], and Cornfield's use of the rare-disease assumption can be seen as stemming from this lack of distinction. Proper methods of adjusting the relative risk estimate were not considered by Cornfield, and his use of adjusted exposure proportion is inadequate. Nevertheless, Cornfield recognized the most serious limitation of his method, namely the possibility of bias in selection of the case and control groups.

Reference:
Vandenbroucke JD. On the rediscovery of a distinction. Am J Epidemiol 1985; 121:627–628.

A METHOD OF ESTIMATING COMPARA-TIVE RATES FROM CLINICAL DATA. APPLICATIONS TO CANCER OF THE LUNG, BREAST, AND CERVIX [1]

JEROME CORNFIELD, *National Cancer Institute, National Institutes of Health, U. S. Public Health Service, Bethesda, Md.*

A frequent problem in epidemiological research is the attempt to determine whether the probability of having or incurring a stated disease, such as cancer of the lung, during a specified interval of time is related to the possession of a certain characteristic, such as smoking. In principle, such a question offers no difficulty. One selects representative groups of persons having and not having the characteristic and determines the percentage in each group who have or develop the disease during this time period. This yields a true rate. The difference in the magnitudes of the rates for those possessing and lacking the characteristic indicates the strength of the association. If it were true, for example, that a very large percentage of cigarette smokers eventually contracted lung cancer, this would suggest the possibility that tobacco is a strong carcinogen.

An investigation that involves selecting representative groups of those having and not having a characteristic is expensive and time consuming, however, and is rarely if ever used. Actual practice in the field is to take two groups presumed to be representative of persons who do and do not have the disease and determine the percentage in each group who have the characteristic. Thus rather than determine the percentage of smokers and nonsmokers who have cancer of the lung, one determines the percentage of persons with and without cancer of the lung who are smokers. This yields, not a true rate, but rather what is usually referred to as a relative frequency. Relative frequencies can be computed with comparative ease from hospital or other clinical records, and in consequence most investigations based on clinical records yield nothing but relative frequencies. The difference in the magnitudes of the relative frequencies does not indicate the strength of the association, however. Even if it were true that there were many more smokers among those with lung cancer than among those without it, this would not by itself suggest whether tobacco was a weak or a strong carcinogen. We are consequently interested in whether it is possible to deduce the rates from knowledge of the relative frequencies.

[1] Received for publication February 23, 1951.

1270   JOURNAL OF THE NATIONAL CANCER INSTITUTE

A GENERAL METHOD

To fix our ideas we may illustrate how the general problem can be attacked with some data recently published by Schrek, Baker, Ballard, and Dolgoff (*1*). They report that 77 percent of the white males studied, aged 40–49, with cancer of the lung, smoked 10 or more cigarettes per day, while only 58 percent of a group of white males, aged 40–49, presumed to be representative of the non-lung-cancer population, smoked that much. Can we estimate from these data the frequency with which cancer of the lung occurs among smokers and nonsmokers?

Denote by p_1 (=0.77) the proportion of smokers among those with cancer of the lung, by p_2 (=0.58) the proportion of smokers among those without cancer of the lung, and by X the proportion of the general population that has cancer of the lung during a specified period of time. We may then summarize the relevant information for the general population in a two-by-two table showing the proportion of the population falling in each of the four possible categories.

Characteristic	Having cancer of the lung	Not having cancer of the lung
Smokers	$p_1 X$	$p_2 (1-X)$
Nonsmokers	$(1-p_1) X$	$(1-p_2) (1-X)$
Total	X	$1-X$

One can now compute that the percentage of the general population that smokes is $p_2 + X(p_1 - p_2)$, that the proportion of smokers having cancer of the lung is:

$$(1)\quad p_1 X / \left[(p_2 + X(p_1 - p_2)) \right].$$

Similarly, the proportion of nonsmokers having cancer of the lung is

$$(2)\quad (1-p_1) X / \left[(1-p_2) - X (p_1 - p_2) \right].$$

Formulas (1) and (2) yield the true rates we seek.

Given the appropriate data, formulas (1) and (2) are easy to compute. They are somewhat cumbersome algebraically, however. The following approximation to the true rates, therefore, seems useful. If the proportion of the general population having cancer of the lung, X, is small relative to both the proportion of the control group smoking and not smoking, p_2 and $1-p_2$, the contribution of the term $X(p_1 - p_2)$ to the denominator of formulas (1) and (2) is trivial and may be neglected. In that case the approximate rate of cancer of the lung among smokers becomes $\dfrac{p_1 X}{p_2}$ and the corresponding rate for nonsmokers $\dfrac{(1-p_1)X}{1-p_2}$. Whenever $p_1 - p_2$ is greater than zero, p_1/p_2 is greater than unity. We may conclude from the approximation, therefore, that whenever a greater proportion of the diseased than of the control group possess a characteristic, the incidence of the disease is always higher among those possessing the characteristic. This is the intuition on which the procedures used in such clinical studies are based. Although it has frequently been questioned, it can now be easily seen to be correct.

It also follows from this analysis, however, that if one knows X, the prevalence of cancer of the lung in the general population, one can compute its prevalence among the smoking and nonsmoking population. Hospital or clinical records usually cannot furnish an estimate of X, however, since one seldom knows the size of the population exposed to risk from which the actual cases are drawn. Its value is frequently known, at least approximately, from other sources. Thus, we have estimated from Dorn's data (2) that the annual prevalence of cancer of the lung among all white males aged 40–49 is 15.5 per 100,000.[2] X consequently is equal to 0.155×10^{-3}. We may now construct a table showing the proportion of the population in each of the four categories from the data of Schrek *et al.*

	Having cancer of the lung	Not having cancer of the lung	Total
Smokers	0.119×10^{-3}	0.579910	0.580029
Nonsmokers	$.036 \times 10^{-3}$	.419935	.419971
Total	$.155 \times 10^{-3}$	.999845	1.000000

The proportion of smokers who have cancer of the lung using formulas (1) and (2) is thus 0.205×10^{-3} as contrasted with 0.086×10^{-3} for nonsmokers. The corresponding rates are 20.5 and 8.6 per 100,000 per year. These rates clearly provide a sounder basis for appraising the effect of cigarette smoking than does the knowledge that 77 percent of those with cancer of the lung and 58 percent without it smoke.

If one is interested only in knowing the relative amount by which the prevalence of the disease is augmented by the possession of the attribute, one may calculate this without knowledge of X, since the ratio of the two rates is $\dfrac{p_1}{p_2} \dfrac{(1-p_2)}{(1-p_1)}$ when X is small. One can thus conclude from the Schrek data alone that the prevalence of cancer of the lung among white males aged 40–49 is 2.4 times as high among those who smoke 10 or more cigarettes a day as among those who do not.

The more extensive, but age-standardized, data of Levin, Goldstein, and Gerhardt (3) on the same subject may be used to illustrate the same calculation. They show that 66.1 percent of all (presumably white) males at all age groups who had cancer of the lung smoked some cigarettes as compared with 44.1 percent smoking among the control group. Setting $.661 = p_1$ and $.441 = p_2$, we have $\dfrac{p_1}{p_2} \dfrac{(1-p_2)}{(1-p_1)} = 2.5$. The prevalence of lung cancer, according to these data is 2.5 times as high among cigarette

---

[2] Dorn's published data show an annual prevalence rate in the period 1937–1939 of 29.7 per 100,000 for cancer of all respiratory organs among white and colored males, aged 40–49. In the North 52.1 percent of the respiratory cases in all age groups for both males and females was accounted for by lung cancer. The estimate of 15.5 (=29.7 × 0.521), is consequently somewhat rough.

smokers as among nonsmokers. (The agreement with the Schrek data is closer than would be expected in view of differences in the population covered, definitions used, and number of cases studied. The application of the present method to other studies of lung cancer and tobacco yields much more divergent results.)

The calculations may also be applied to multiple classifications such as the data on cancer of the cervix in Cardiff, Wales, recently published by Maliphant (4). In table 1, the first column gives the percent distribution of women who develop cancer of the cervix by marital status and number of children borne, while the second column shows the same distribution for all women. Women under 40 have been excluded. From other data given by Maliphant we have estimated that the incidence rate of cervical cancer for women over 40 in Cardiff was 79.7 per 100,000 (somewhat below the corresponding rate in this country.) This yields X and we accordingly have been able to calculate the incidence rates by marital status and number of children shown in the third column. The relation between cervical cancer and number of children born is obviously shown more clearly and usefully by the rates in the third column than by the relative frequencies in the first two.

TABLE 1.—*Distribution of women with and without cervical cancer by marital status and number of children*

	Women contracting cancer of the cervix, 100 p_1	All women, 100 p_2	Incidence rate per 100,000, $\dfrac{p_1 X}{p_2}$
Unmarried	1.3	10.5	9.9
Married:			
No children	5.0	13.0	30.7
1 or more children, total	93.7	76.5	97.6
1 child	13.3	15.3	69.3
2 children	18.3	17.0	85.8
3 children	15.0	13.0	92.0
4 children	11.0	9.6	91.3
5 children	9.2	6.4	114.6
6 or more	26.9	15.2	141.6
Total	100.0	100.0	

TESTS OF SIGNIFICANCE ON THE COMPUTED RATE

Since most clinical studies are based on limited numbers of cases, it is of some importance to be able to estimate the limits of error of rates calculated according to this procedure. The approximate formula for the variance of a ratio sometimes used is inappropriate for this purpose, since it will sometimes show $\dfrac{p_2 X}{p_1}$ differing significantly from X when a test on the difference $p_2\text{-}p_1$ shows that it does not differ significantly from zero. To avoid this we employ a test of Fieller's (5). Thus, writing the computed prevalence rate as $\dfrac{p_1 X}{p_2}=r$ and denoting by

$n_1=$ the number of disease cases

$n_2 =$ the number of control cases

$t_\alpha =$ the value of t in the normal curve corresponding to the 100α-percent probability level

$pq =$ the unbiased estimate of the unknown population value PQ

$$\left(= \frac{n_1 p_1 + n_2 p_2}{n_1 + n_2 - 1} \left[1 - \frac{n_1 p_1 + n_2 p_2}{n_1 + n_2} \right] \right)$$

the upper and lower confidence limits for the 100α-percent probability level of the estimate r are given by

$$\frac{r \pm \dfrac{t_\alpha X}{p_2} \sqrt{\dfrac{pq}{n_1} \left[1 + \dfrac{1}{n_2 p_2{}^2} (n_1 p_1^2 - t_\alpha^2 pq) \right]^{\frac{1}{2}}}}{1 - \dfrac{t_\alpha{}^2 pq}{n_2 p_2{}^2}},$$

when X is considered free from sampling error. We may use the Schrek data to illustrate the use of this formula. Thus, letting $n_1 = 35$, $n_2 = 171$, setting $t_\alpha = 2$, and using p, X, and r as previously calculated, we compute the upper limit to the rate as 25.6 per 100,000 and the lower limit as 16.1 per 100,000. Since the value of X used, 15.5 per 100,000, falls outside these limits, we conclude that the rates for smokers and nonsmokers differ significantly at the 5-percent probability level. Whenever p_1 and p_2 differ significantly at the 100α-percent level, the limits computed in this fashion will not include X, and *vice versa*. Thus, if one simply wishes to test significance, it is sufficient to test the difference between p_1 and p_2. If one wishes to express error limits in the same units that the prevalence rate is expressed, however, one must use the formula given.[3]

PITFALLS

Our major purpose in preparing this note has been to show that any set of data that furnishes estimates of relative frequencies can be used to obtain estimates of rates. The procedure suggested, however, has assumed that the diseased and control groups used are representative of these same groups in the general population. If this assumption is not satisfied, then neither the rates, the relative frequencies, nor any other statistics calculated from the data will have applicability beyond the particular group studied.

We may illustrate the difficulties that can arise on this score with 2 examples. The first relates to Lane-Claypon's study of cancer of the breast (*6*). In this study a detailed questionnaire was filled in for 508

---

[3] The procedure discussed in the text yields a two-sided test of significance; i. e., it tests the hypothesis that the rate for smokers is significantly different from that for nonsmokers. It would be more realistic to use a one-sided test; i. e., test the hypothesis that the rate for smokers is significantly *higher* than that for nonsmokers. To do this one uses the same formula but calculates only a lower limit, using a value of t_α appropriate to the one-sided test. Thus, for $\alpha = 0.05$, $t_\alpha = 1.645$.

In testing whether p_1 and p_2 are drawn from the same population it is appropriate to compute a pooled variance as has been done. When the results of such a test of significance suggest that p_1 and p_2 could not have been drawn from the same population, however, the use of a pooled variance to compute error limits is no longer correct. In fact, exact confidence limits can no longer be calculated for this case. The results yielded by the formula will nevertheless be sufficiently accurate for most practical purposes.

women with breast cancer and 509 control women, who were being treated by the cooperating hospitals for "some trouble, other than cancer." We reproduce in table 2 the percent distribution by number of children ever borne for each group. Only women having passed the menopause are included. We do not know X, the prevalence rate of breast cancer in the United Kingdom at the time the data were collected, and have therefore confined ourselves to computing relative prevalence.

TABLE 2.—*Distribution of women with and without breast cancer by marital status and number of children*

Characteristic	Cancer group, p_1	Control group, p_2	$\frac{p_1}{p_2}$	Relative prevalence
Unmarried	20. 91	16. 42	1. 273	100
Married:				
No children	14. 55	10. 45	1. 392	109
1 to 3 children	29. 09	24. 78	1. 174	92
4 to 6 children	21. 21	22. 39	. 947	74
7 or more	14. 24	25. 97	. 548	43
Total	100. 00	100. 00		

If the data are to be taken at their face value, one must conclude that lowered prevalence of breast cancer is associated with increasing numbers of children. Greenwood in an analysis of Lane-Claypon's data (6) in fact concludes, "we think then that an etiological factor of importance has now been fully demonstrated." At the very beginning of his analysis, however, he points out, without attaching any significance to it, that the control group had borne an average of about 25 percent more children than had all women in England and Wales with the same duration of marriage. This would appear to provide definite evidence for the unrepresentative character of the control group and to cast doubt on the adequacy of the evidence.

The basic difficulty in this example is the unrepresentative nature of the control group. Since there is always some doubt whether or not a control group selected from among hospital patients can provide an accurate estimate of the frequency of a characteristic in the population at large, the difficulty may be quite general. The possibility that the diseased group is not representative either, cannot be entirely disregarded, however. We reproduce in table 3 the distribution by age of 413 patients with adenocarcinoma of the breast admitted to the Ellis Fischel State Cancer Hospital in the years 1940–46 as given by Ackerman and Regato (7). For comparison we give the expected distribution on the basis of known incidence rates by age.

It is obvious from inspection that an excess number in the older age groups were encountered, and that to some extent the hospital was functioning as a home for the aged. An epidemiological investigation the results of which would be sensitive to the age distribution of the persons studied might consequently be adversely affected.

Any set of hospital or clinical data that is worth analyzing at all is

COMPARATIVE RATE FROM CLINICAL DATA   1275

TABLE 3.—*Actual and expected distribution of breast cancer cases by age—Ellis Fischel State Cancer Hospital*

| Age | Number of breast cancer cases [1] | | (3) (4) × (5) | Incidence of breast cancer per 100,000 [2] (4) | Percent distribution Missouri population 1940 [3] (5) |
	Reported (1)	Expected (2) (3) $\frac{\text{Tot. (1)}}{\text{Tot. (3)}}$			
Less than 30	3	7	1. 1	2. 2	0. 4825
30–34	10	13	1. 9	25. 1	. 0795
35–39	24	25	3. 7	50. 7	. 0774
40–44	26	41	6. 1	91. 1	. 0734
45–49	40	54	8. 0	122. 9	. 0674
50–54	51	51	7. 5	129. 0	. 0648
55–59	54	57	8. 4	169. 6	. 0580
60–64	54	53	7. 8	190. 4	. 0495
65–69	59	45	6. 6	193. 3	. 0410
70–74	48	34	5. 1	205. 5	. 0344
75 and over	44	33	4. 9	184. 5	. 0516
Total	413	413	61. 1		1. 0000

[1] Chi square for difference = 24.5, $P < 0.01$.
[2] As estimated by Dorn (*2*).
[3] U. S. Bureau of the Census, Population, vol. II, pt. 4, table 7.

worth analyzing properly. It is from this point of view that the technique proposed seems useful. The preceding two examples suggest, however, that the results of even the most carefully analyzed set of such data may be open to question, and that these doubts can be resolved only by methods of data collection that provide representative samples of diseased and nondiseased persons.

REFERENCES

(*1*) SCHREK, R., BAKER, L. A., BALLARD, G. P., and DOLGOFF, S.: Tobacco smoking as an etiologic factor in disease. I. Cancer. Cancer Research 10: 49–58, 1950.

(*2*) DORN, H. F.: Illness from cancer in the United States. Pub. Health Rep. 59, Nos. 2, 3 and 4, 1944.

(*3*) LEVIN, M. L., GOLDSTEIN, H., and GERHARDT, P. R.: Cancer and tobacco smoking. J. A. M. A. 143: 336–338, 1950.

(*4*) MALIPHANT, R. G.: The incidence of cancer of the uterine cervix. Brit. M. J., I: 978–982, 1949.

(*5*) FIELLER, E. C.: The biological standardization of insulin. Supp. J. Roy. Stat. Soc. 7: 1–64, 1940.

(*6*) LANE-CLAYPON, J. E.: A further report on cancer of the breast. Reports on Public Health and Medical Subjects, No. 32, Ministry of Health, London, 1926.

(*7*) ACKERMAN, L. V., and del REGATO, J. A.: Cancer, Diagnosis, Treatment and Prognosis. C. V. Mosby Co., St. Louis, 1947, p. 927.

II–3.

E. H. Simpson: The Interpretation of Interaction in Contingency Tables. Journal of the Royal Statistical Society 1951; B13:238–241.

Simpson's "The Interpretation of Interaction in Contingency Tables" is probably better known among statisticians than epidemiologists, so its importance may be more indirect than the other articles presented here. Nevertheless, it is a landmark in its consideration of the perils associated with the concepts of interaction and collapsibility in contingency tables. It was Simpson who noted the difficulties of translating commonsense notions of statistical interaction into a precise mathematical form, in particular the fact that one's impression of the presence or absence of interaction depends on one's choice of measure of association (see paragraph 3 of the article). He also noted what, for a time at least, was known as "Simpson's paradox": that one's chosen measure of association between two variables may be identical within levels of a third variable, but may take on an entirely different value when the third variable is ignored, i.e., when the levels of the third variable are "collapsed" to form a single "crude" table. Epidemiologists will recognize this in the all-too-familiar problem of confounding, although Simpson also noted that in some cases — when the third variable is irrelevant – the crude measure is the appropriate one. For the record, one should note that the so-called "paradox" was clearly described by Yule [1903] a half-century before Simpson.

For the binary-variable case that he considered, Simpson showed that for his "paradox" to occur, it was necessary and sufficient for the third variable to be associated with both of the two variables of interest. It was some 27 years before Whittemore [1978] showed that the sufficiency of the latter condition held only if the third variable was binary. That is, if the third variable had more than two levels, it was possible for it to be associated with the other two variables and yet the crude and specific associations could still be equal. The only other point overlooked by Simpson that I could discern was in paragraph 5. Here Simpson failed to note that the fatality rate difference does satisfy an important symmetry property: the interaction of the rate difference will be of the same magnitude no matter which of the two antecedent variables is considered the treatment variable. The more general three-attribute symmetry property (given in paragraph 3) is, as Simpson notes, possessed by the odds ratio but not the rate difference; however, it is not a necessity when dealing with measures of effect.

References:
Whittemore AS. Collapsibility of multidimensional contingency tables. J Roy Statist Soc Ser B 1978; 40:328–340.
Yule GU. Notes on the theory of association of attributes in statistics. Biometrika 1903; 2:121–134, section 6.

238   [No. 2.

THE INTERPRETATION OF INTERACTION IN CONTINGENCY TABLES

By E. H. SIMPSON

[Received May, 1951]

SUMMARY

THE definition of second order interaction in a $(2 \times 2 \times 2)$ table given by Bartlett is accepted, but it is shown by an example that the vanishing of this second order interaction does not necessarily justify the mechanical procedure of forming the three component 2×2 tables and testing each of these for significance by standard methods.*

1. In a $2 \times 2 \times 2$ contingency table in which each entry is classified according to its possession or not of each of three attributes, there may exist not only associations or interactions of these attributes in pairs, but also a second order interaction of all three taken together. Bartlett (1935) has outlined a test for the presence of such a second order interaction, and Norton (1945) has discussed the numerical processes involved in carrying it out. The purpose of this note is to examine more fully the meaning of the test and its interpretation in practical examples.

2. Suppose a $2 \times 2 \times 2$ table is made up by classifying entries according to their possession of the attributes A or $\overline{A}$, B or $\overline{B}$, C or $\overline{C}$, where as usual $\overline{A}$ denotes "not-A" and so on, and let $a, b, \ldots h$ be the probabilities that an entry will fall in one of the eight classes so formed, thus:

TABLE 1

	CB	$C\overline{B}$	$\overline{C}B$	$\overline{C}\,\overline{B}$
A . . .	a	c	e	g
$\overline{A}$ . . .	b	d	f	h

Obviously $a + b + c + d + e + f + g + h = 1$.

The extension to this case of the hypothesis of independence which is commonly applied to the 2×2 table, namely that the probability of the class AB is the product of the probabilities of the classes A and B, gives us equations of the form

$$a = (a + c + e + g)(a + b + e + f)(a + b + c + d).$$

This is the statement of the hypothesis of complete independence of the three attributes, and any given experimental data could be tested on it by calculating the theoretical cell contents from the totals of A, of B and of C in the total sample and forming a χ^2 which would have 4 degrees of freedom.

---

* This paper should be read in conjunction with the following paper by H. O. Lancaster. Bartlett's condition for a zero second order interaction is (in Simpson's notation)

$$\binom{a}{b} \Big/ \binom{c}{d} = \binom{e}{f} \Big/ \binom{g}{h}.$$

Lancaster defines the second order interaction so as to make χ^2 additive. In general his χ^2 component for interaction is different from Bartlett's, but he shows that they are asymptotically the same. On Lancaster's definition the condition for zero second order interaction is

$$a(q\, q'\, q'') - b(p\, q'\, p'') - c(q\, p'\, q'') + d(p\, p'\, q'') - e(q\, q'\, p'') + f(p\, q'\, p'') + g(q\, p'\, p'') - h(p\, p'\, p'')$$

where

$$p = (a + c + e + g)/N, \qquad p' = (a + b + e + f)/N, \qquad p'' = (a + b + c + d)/N.$$

This satisfies the condition of symmetry mentioned by Simpson.—ED.

3. The four degrees of freedom of χ^2 suggest that there are four ways in which the cell probabilities can depart from complete independence, and it is reasonable to associate with them the three first order interactions, A with B, B with C, C with A, and something which we shall call the second order interaction. So far it is open to us to define as we like the boundary between first order and second order interaction, since no definition of the latter is forced upon us by what has gone before. Common sense suggests some statement such as this:

> "Granting that there is an association between the attributes A and B, we shall say that there is no second order interaction between A and B on the one hand and C on the other if the degree of association between A and B is the same in the class C as it is in the class $\overline{C}$."

This is a rather more general statement than that given by Norton (1939). Two difficulties immediately present themselves:

(i) We now require to measure the degree of association of two attributes in a 2×2 table. Various measures have been suggested (see for instance Kendall (1945), chapter 13), and it is reasonable to expect the use of different measures in the simple table to lead to different definitions of second order interaction in the more complex one.

(ii) The above statement is not symmetrical in all three attributes. We could similarly define the absence of second order interaction between B-and-C and A, and between C-and-A and B. Should the three sets of conditions be identical?

If on consideration of (ii) we decide that our definition of "no second order interaction" should be symmetrical with respect to the three attributes, and this is a logically attractive condition, then the choice of measures under (i) will be considerably restricted. For if in Table 1 we choose some function $\psi(a, b, c, d)$ to measure the association of A and B in the class C, the function must be such that the equation

$$\psi(a, b, c, d) = \psi(e, f, g, h)$$

implies and is implied by the equations

$$\psi(a, c, e, g) = \psi(b, d, f, h) \text{ and } \psi(a, b, e, f) = \psi(c, d, g, h).$$

This condition of symmetry is not satisfied, for instance, by the root mean square contingency defined by

$$\frac{ad - bc}{\{(a + b)(a + c)(b + d)(c + d)\}^{\frac{1}{2}}}.$$

But it is satisfied by $\psi = bc/ad$, which was used in rather similar circumstances by Fisher (1935), page 50, and by any simple function of bc/ad such as the coefficient of association

$$Q = (1 - bc/ad) \div (1 + bc/ad)$$

or the coefficient of colligation

$$Y = (1 - \sqrt{bc/ad}) \div (1 + \sqrt{bc/ad}).$$

If we use either bc/ad, Q or Y as our measure, the definition of absence of second order interaction becomes

$$adfg = bceh,$$

which is the form of the hypothesis stated by Bartlett (1935).

4. In order to obtain a clearer notion of the assumptions underlying this Bartlett test let us take an example in which, as is often the case, B and C are treatments applied to a patient of some kind, A is the classification "alive" and $\overline{A}$ the classification "dead". To describe the fatality in each of the treatment classes we shall use, not the conventional fatality rate, but the ratio of deaths to survivals. The effect of a treatment is to multiply this ratio by some factor which will be less than unity if the treatment is beneficial. Referring back to Table 1, the ratio in the untreated class $\overline{BC}$ is h/g, that in the class treated by B alone is f/e and that in the class treated by C alone

is d/c, and so the factors associated with B and C are fg/eh and dg/ch respectively. The combination of treatments BC has a factor bg/ah, and the condition for no second order interaction, $adfg = bceh$, is seen at once to be the same as

$$\frac{bg}{ah} = \frac{fg}{eh}\frac{dg}{ch},$$

that is, the factor for treatment BC is the product of the factors for B and C alone. In other words, the effect of treatment B is to multiply the dead/alive ratio by the same factor whatever other treatments may have been used; and similarly for treatment C.

5. Returning to our contingency table, it is of interest to notice the consequences of thinking in terms of fatality rates instead of the dead/alive ratio. In an example quoted by Norton (1939) the classes C and $\bar{C}$ are male and female animals, B is a treatment, and A is "alive". Norton then states that to test for second order interaction we find the difference in death rates between "controls" (untreated) and "experimentals" (treated) and compare the values of the difference in the male and female categories. In the notation of Table 1 this gives as the condition for the absence of second order interaction

$$\frac{b}{a+b} - \frac{d}{c+d} = \frac{f}{e+f} - \frac{h}{g+h}$$

or

$$\frac{bc - ad}{(a+b)(c+d)} = \frac{fg - eh}{(e+f)(g+h)}.$$

This is equivalent to taking as a measure of association in a 2×2 table

$$\frac{bc - ad}{(a+b)(c+d)},$$

which does not satisfy the symmetry condition.

6. Let us now consider the interpretation to be placed on the three first order interactions in the two cases when second order interaction does or does not exist.

7. If second order interaction does exist, the course of action is clear but dull. No two classifications can be said to be independent, for if, say, A and B are independent in C, then by hypothesis they cannot be independent in $\bar{C}$. In general it is impossible to summarize the relationship of any two classifications without reference to the third, and the only course is to set out the six possible 2×2 tables and enumerate the relationsips of A and B in C, of A and B in $\bar{C}$, and so on.

8. If, however, there is no second order interaction, there is considerable scope for paradox and error. The dangers of amalgamating 2×2 tables are well known and are referred to, for example, on page 317 of Kendall (1945), vol. I. Kendall's example illustrates that if A and B are associated positively in C and negatively in $\bar{C}$ they may appear as independent in the whole population; but a more curious case than this can be constructed. Consider the following artificial example.

9. An investigator wished to examine whether in a pack of cards the proportion of court cards (King, Queen, Knave) was associated with colour. It happened that the pack which he examined was one with which Baby had been playing, and some of the cards were dirty. He included the classification "dirty" in his scheme in case it was relevant, and obtained the following probabilities:

TABLE 2

	Dirty		Clean	
	Court	Plain	Court	Plain
Red . . .	4/52	8/52	2/52	12/52
Black . . .	3/52	5/52	3/52	15/52

It will be observed that Baby preferred red cards to black and court cards to plain, but showed

no second order interaction on Bartlett's definition. The investigator deduced a positive association between redness and plainness both among the dirty cards and among the clean, yet it is
the combined table

TABLE 3

	Court	Plain
Red . . .	6/52	20/52
Black . . .	6/52	20/52

which provides what we would call the sensible answer, namely, that there is no such association.
   10. Suppose we now change the names of the classes in Table 2 thus:

TABLE 4

	Male		Female	
	Untreated	*Treated*	*Untreated*	*Treated*
Alive . . .	4/52	8/52	2/52	12/52
Dead . . .	3/52	5/52	3/52	15/52

The probabilities are exactly the same as in Table 2, and there is again the same degree of positive
association in each of the 2 × 2 tables. This time we say that there is a positive association
between treatment and survival both among males and among females; but if we combine the
tables we again find that there is no association between treatment and survival in the combined
population. What is the "sensible" interpretation here? The treatment can hardly be rejected
as valueless to the race when it is beneficial when applied to males and to females.
   11. It is sometimes said—for example in Norton (1939) and on page 203 of Snedecor (1946)—
that provided there is no second order interaction it is permissible to add a 2 × 2 × 2 table in
each of the three possible ways and to test for independence in the resulting three 2 × 2 tables.
The example just given shows that this is false. What can be said is that, assuming there is no
second order interaction, the degree of association in the combined table (measured by ψ) will
be the same as that in the separate tables C and $\overline{C}$ if and only if the classification C which is being
submerged is independent either of A in both B and $\overline{B}$ or of B in both A and $\overline{A}$. For suppose
that in Table 1 there is no second order interaction, so that $bc/ad = fg/eh$, and that the two 2 × 2
tables in C and $\overline{C}$ respectively are combined in the ratio 1 : λ. If the resulting table is to show the
same degree of association between A and B we must have

$$\frac{(b + \lambda f)(c + \lambda g)}{(a + \lambda e)(d + \lambda h)} = \frac{bc}{ad} = \frac{fg}{eh},$$

which reduces to

$$\lambda(af - be)(ag - ce)h/a = 0.$$

Thus (trivial cases apart) no linear combination of the tables will preserve the value of the association unless either $af = be$ or $ag = ce$, which represent respectively the conditions that C and A
are independent in B (and consequently also in $\overline{B}$ though not necessarily in the whole population)
and that C and B are independent in A. Kendall's statement that if A and B are independent
in both C and $\overline{C}$ they are not independent in the population as a whole unless C is independent
of A or B or both is a special case of this rule.
   12. I am indebted to Professor M. S. Bartlett for having suggested, some years ago now, that
this subject needed further consideration.

References

BARTLETT, M. S. (1935), *J. R. Statist. Soc. Suppl.*, **2**, 248.
FISHER, R. A. (1935), *J. R. Statist. Soc.*, **98**, 39.
KENDALL, M. G. (1945), *The Advanced Theory of Statistics*, vol. I. Griffin.
NORTON, H. W. (1939), *Brit. Med. Journ.*, **2**, 467.
—— (1945), *J. Amer. Statist. Ass.*, **40**, 251.
SNEDECOR, G. W. (1946), *Statistical Methods*. Iowa State College Press.

II–4.

Barnet Woolf: On Estimating the Relation Between Blood Group and Disease. Annals of Human Genetics 1955; 19:251–253.

Woolf's "On Estimating the Relation Between Blood Group and Disease" is most often cited for its introduction of what was probably the first common odds-ratio estimator for a set of two-by-two tables (or studies), and a test for heterogeneity of the odds ratio across the tables; these are now known as Woolf's estimate and Woolf's test of homogeneity (see, e.g., Schlesselman [1982]). Though these statistics have been supplanted by Mantel-Haenszel and maximum-likelihood methods, the paper contains more than just bare mechanics, as it touches on a number of important points which were generally unappreciated in the early literature.

Woolf was motivated by concern about the then-prevalent practice of analyzing and comparing case-control results by computing the difference in exposure proportions between case and control groups. As he notes, this difference would vary with the background frequency of exposure, and artifactual differences between study results could be expected. Instead he chose to work with the ratio of incidence rates, and recognized (independently of Cornfield) that this ratio could be estimated from case-control data, even if the absolute rates could not. (He did not, however, delineate sufficient conditions for the sample odds ratio to estimate the incidence ratio.) He also noted some subtle points that many later users of his methods overlooked, one being that his variance formula for the common odds ratio applied only under the homogeneity assumption.

Reference:
Schlesselman JJ. *Case-control Studies: Design, Conduct, Analysis.* New York: Oxford University Press, 1982.

[251]

ON ESTIMATING THE RELATION BETWEEN BLOOD GROUP AND DISEASE

By BARNET WOOLF

Department of Animal Genetics, University of Edinburgh

Following the demonstration of a significant excess of blood group A in patients with cancer of the stomach (Aird, Bentall & Roberts, 1953) and of group O in sufferers from peptic ulcer (Aird, Bentall, Mehigan & Roberts, 1954) and from toxaemia of pregnancy (Pike & Dickins, 1954) it seems certain that many more studies will be made on the relation between blood groups and disease. It is therefore important that the best possible statistical methods should be used. The procedure recommended by Aird *et al.* (1954) is very efficient, but it is open to criticism on one rather important point. These workers take as criterion the difference in proportion of a given blood group in the disease and the control series. Denote the two blood types α and β. Suppose the disease series contains h patients of type α and k of type β, where $h + k = n$, and the control series has H of type α and K of type β, where $H + K = N$. Aird and associates calculate $d = h/n - H/N$. This is tested for significance against its sampling variance, combined with estimates from other bodies of data to give a weighted mean estimate, and compared with these other estimates in tests for heterogeneity.

Unfortunately, d will differ from one community to another even when the specific attack rate within any given blood group stays constant. This can be shown by a simple example. Consider a community of 10,000 people in which H and K are each 5000. Then if $h = 100$ and $k = 50$, $d = 100/150 - 0.5$, or 0.1667. Now consider another community in which H is 9000 and K is 1000. In this case $h = 180$ and $k = 10$, so $d = 180/190 - 0.9$, or 0.0474. Even when the essential biological conditions are identical, differences in blood-group frequencies in the population will introduce spurious heterogeneity. This kind of artefact is avoided if one works with incidence rates in the various blood groups. The data usually do not permit calculation of absolute rates, nor are they needed. What is wanted and readily obtained is an estimate of the ratio of one rate to another. The incidence in group α will be $h/H \times$ some constant, and that in group β will be $k/K \times$ the same constant. If the ratio is taken as x to 1, an estimate of x will be hK/Hk, and it may readily be shown that this is the maximum-likelihood estimate. The use of x is recommended instead of d as a criterion of differential incidence of disease in relation to blood group.

In all statistical computations it is best to transform x into its logarithm. This avoids difficulties due to asymmetry. If comparison of α with β gives $x = 2$ say, comparison of β with α will give $x = \frac{1}{2}$; but $\log x$ will retain its numerical value, merely changing in sign. Moreover, the sampling variance of $\log x$ is a very simple expression free of 'nuisance parameters'. This is especially true if one transforms into $y = \log_e x$. If V is the sampling variance of y, then

$$V = 1/h + 1/k + 1/H + 1/K,$$

and w, the weight of y, is of course $1/V$. If the attack rate is the same for both blood types the expected value of y will be 0, so the null hypothesis is not to be rejected unless y differs significantly from zero. This is tested by χ^2 will be y^2/V or wy^2 for one degree of freedom. Combination of data from different communities proceeds as described by Aird *et al.* (1954). The weighted mean, Y,

BLOOD GROUP AND DISEASE

is $\Sigma wy/\Sigma w$, and its antilogarithm, X, is taken as the combined estimate of x. Significance of Y is tested by $\chi^2 = (\Sigma wy)^2/\Sigma w$ or $Y^2\Sigma w$ for one degree of freedom. Heterogeneity is tested by $\chi^2 = \Sigma wy^2 - (\Sigma wy)^2/\Sigma w$ or $\Sigma wy^2 - Y^2\Sigma w$ with degrees of freedom one less than the number of sets of data combined. The standard deviation of y is $V^{\frac{1}{2}}$, and the approximate fiducial limits at the 95 % point are $y \pm 1.96 V^{\frac{1}{2}}$. Provided there is no significant heterogeneity the standard deviation of Y is $1/(\Sigma w)^{\frac{1}{2}}$ and the 95 % fiducial limits are approximately $Y \pm 1.96/(\Sigma w)^{\frac{1}{2}}$. By taking antilogarithms these can be transformed into fiducial limits for x or X. This is a 'large-sample' treatment, and the formulae cease to be applicable if any of the observed frequencies is small.

Table 1. *Calculation of combined estimate of incidence ratio of peptic ulcer in groups O and A*

| City | Peptic ulcer | | Control | | $x=\dfrac{hK}{Hk}$ | $y=\log_e x$ | $w=\dfrac{1}{\dfrac{1}{h}+\dfrac{1}{k}+\dfrac{1}{H}+\dfrac{1}{K}}$ | $wy^2=\chi^2$ |
	Group O (h)	Group A (k)	Group O (H)	Group A (K)				
London	911	579	4578	4219	1.4500	0.3716	304.9	42.11
Manchester	361	246	4532	3775	1.2224	0.2008	136.6	5.50
Newcastle	396	219	6598	5261	1.4418	0.3659	134.5	18.01
					$\Sigma wy = 189.94$		576.0	65.62

$Y = \Sigma wy/\Sigma w = 0.3289$.
$Y^2\Sigma w = 62.63$.
s.d. of $Y = (\Sigma w)^{-\frac{1}{2}} = 0.0417$.
95 % fiducial limits of $Y = 0.2472 - 0.4106$.
$X = $ antilog $Y = 1.39$.
95 % fiducial limits of $X = 1.28 - 1.51$.

χ^2 analysis

	D.F.	
Y	1	62.63
Heterogeneity	2	2.99
Total	3	65.62

Table 2. *Incidence ratios of some diseases in relation to blood group*

Disease	Comparison	X or x	95 % fiducial limits	Reference
Cancer of stomach	Group A with group O	1.22	1.12–1.32	Aird et al. (1953)
Peptic ulcer	Group O with group A	1.39	1.28–1.51	Aird et al. (1954)
Toxaemia of pregnancy	Group O with all others	1.38	1.15–1.66	Pike & Dickins (1954)

Table 1 shows the calculations for comparing incidence of peptic ulcer in groups O and A using combined data from London, Manchester and Newcastle. This is the example worked out by their method by Aird et al. (1954, Table VII). The χ^2 values, 62.63 for significance and 2.99 for heterogeneity, agree closely with 66.21 and 3.01 found by the d method. Similarly, combined data from six centres on cancer of the stomach in groups O and A gave χ^2 values by the x method of 21.28 (1 D.F.) for significance and 2.63 (5 D.F.) for heterogeneity, against 21.49 and 2.69 by the d method. These close concordances are to be expected, since the observations all come from cities in England with very similar population blood-group frequencies. If data from different ethnic groups were combined, the d method would in general be expected to return unduly high χ^2 figures for heterogeneity. This might be of some biological or medical importance as tending to be confounded with possible genuine heterogeneity arising either from environmental factors or from differential attack rates for the diverse genotypes that may go to make up a single blood group. Even when heterogeneity is not an issue, x is preferable to d because it has a direct medical meaning. Table 2 gives some estimated incidence ratios of diseases in relation to blood group, together with fiducial limits. A blood-group difference appears able to increase the risk of disease by as much as 39 %.

REFERENCES

AIRD, I., BENTALL, H. H., MEHIGAN, J. A. & ROBERTS, J. A. F. (1954). The blood groups in relation to peptic ulceration and carcinoma of colon, rectum, breast and bronchus. *Brit. Med. J.* **2**, 315.

AIRD, I., BENTALL, H. H. & ROBERTS, J. A. F. (1953). The relationship beteeen cancer of stomach and the *ABO* blood groups. *Brit. Med. J.* **1**, 799.

PIKE, L. A. & DICKINS, A. M. (1954). *ABO* blood groups and toxaemia of pregnancy. *Brit. Med. J.* **2**, 321.

II–5.

Nathan Mantel and William Haenszel: Statistical Aspects of the Analysis of Data From Retrospective Studies of Disease. Journal of The National Cancer Institute 1959; 22:719–748.

Mantel and Haenszel's "Statistical Aspects of the Analysis of Data from Retrospective Studies of Disease" is justly famous for its introduction of the test and estimator of a common odds ratio named after the authors. But this paper, by far the longest in this collection, discussed much more than formulas: it also reviewed the history and theory of case-control studies as they stood before 1959. Along with Cornfield and Haenszel's "Some aspects of retrospective studies" [1960] and Dorn's "Some problems arising in prospective and retrospective studies of the etiology of disease" [1959], it long served as text material for basic coursework on case-control studies (indeed, these papers were still in service when I began studying epidemiology). In this regard it may be of interest only in contrast to modern theory: for example, Mantel and Haenszel emphasize on page 722 that

> "A primary goal is to reach the same conclusion in a retrospective study as would have been obtained from a forward study, if one had been done."

This has (hopefully) been replaced by an objective common to all studies of obtaining *valid* results, in clearer recognition that "forward" studies (even randomized ones) are also subject to bias. Nevertheless, many concerns have not changed, such as those regarding hospital-based studies.

On the purely statistical side, the Mantel-Haenszel odds ratio is a fascinating item. The authors arrived at it solely through very informal considerations and contrasts against possible alternatives, yet after more than two decades of study the estimator was found to be nearly as optimal in performance as far more complicated procedures, and much better than some long-standing competitors (such as the Woolf estimator, discussed in the preceding paper) [Breslow, 1981]. The Mantel-Haenszel test meanwhile was extended by Mantel to ordinal data and failure-time (survival) analysis [Mantel, 1963, and 1966]; in the latter case it is now better known as the log-rank test. The test has also been shown to have certain large-sample optimality properties [Gart and Tarone, 1983].

References:
Breslow N. Odds ratio estimators when the data are sparse. Biometrika 1981; 68:73–84.
Cornfield J, Haenszel, WH. Some aspects of retrospective studies. J Chron Dis 1960; 11:523–534.
Dorn HF. Some problems arising in prospective and retrospective studies of the etiology of disease. N Eng J Med 1959; 261:571–579.
Gart JJ, Tarone RE. The relation between score tests and approximate UMPU tests in experimental models common in biometry. Biometrics 1983; 39:781–786.
Mantel N. Chi-square tests with one degree of freedom: extensions of the Mantel-Haenszel procedure. J Am Statist Assoc 1963; 99:129–138.
Mantel N. Evaluation of survival data and two new rank order statistics arising in its consideration. Cancer Chem Rep 1966; 50:163–170.

Statistical Aspects of the Analysis of Data From Retrospective Studies of Disease [1]

Nathan Mantel *and* William Haenszel, *Biometry Branch, National Cancer Institute,* [2] *Bethesda, Maryland*

Summary

The role and limitations of retrospective investigations of factors possibly associated with the occurrence of a disease are discussed and their relationship to forward-type studies emphasized. Examples of situations in which misleading associations could arise through the use of inappropriate control groups are presented. The possibility of misleading associations may be minimized by controlling or matching on factors which could produce such associations; the statistical analysis will then be modified. Statistical methodology is presented for analyzing retrospective study data, including chi-square measures of statistical significance of the observed association between the disease and the factor under study, and measures for interpreting the association in terms of an increased relative risk of disease. An extension of the chi-square test to the situation where data are subclassified by factors controlled in the analysis is given. A summary relative risk formula, R, is presented and discussed in connection with the problem of weighting the individual subcategory relative risks according to their importance or their precision. Alternative relative-risk formulas, R_1, R_2, R_3, and R_4, which require the calculation of subcategory-adjusted proportions of the study factor among diseased persons and controls for the computation of relative risks, are discussed. While these latter formulas may be useful in many instances, they may be biased or inconsistent and are not, in fact, averages of the relative risks observed in the separate subcategories. Only the relative-risk formula, R, of those presented, can be viewed as such an average. The relationship of the matched-sample method to the subclassification approach is indicated. The statistical methodology presented is illustrated with examples from a study of women with epidemoid and undifferentiated pulmonary carcinoma.—J. Nat. Cancer Inst. 22: 719–748, 1959.

Introduction

A retrospective study of disease occurrence may be defined as one in which the determination of association of a disease with some factor is based on an unusually high or low frequency of that factor among diseased persons. This contrasts with a forward study in which one looks instead

[1] Received for publication November 6, 1958.
[2] National Institutes of Health, Public Health Service, U.S. Department of Health, Education, and Welfare.

719

for an unusually high or low occurrence of the disease among individuals possessing the factor in question. Each approach has its advantages. Among the desirable attributes of the retrospective study is the ability to yield results from presently collectible data, whereas the forward study usually requires future observation of individuals over an extended period (this is not always true; if the status of individuals can be determined as of some past date, the data for a forward study may already be at hand). The retrospective approach is also adapted to the limited resources of an individual investigator and places a premium on the formulation of hypotheses for testing, rather than on facilities for data collection. For especially rare diseases a retrospective study may be the only feasible approach, since the forward study may prove too expensive to consider and the study size required to obtain a respectable number of cases completely unmanageable.

In the absence of important biases in the study setting, the retrospective method could be regarded, according to sound statistical theory, as the study method of choice. This follows from the much reduced sample sizes required by this approach and may be illustrated by the following extreme example. If a disease attack rate of 10 per 100,000 among 50 percent of the population free of some factor were increased tenfold among the other half of the population subject to the factor, a retrospective study of 100 cases and 100 controls would, with high probability, reveal this significantly increased risk. On the other hand, a forward study covering 2,000 persons, half with and half without the factor, would almost certainly fail to detect a significant difference. For comparable ability to find the type of increased risk just indicated, a forward study would need to cover about 500 times as many individuals as the corresponding retrospective study. The disparity in the required number of persons to be studied could, of course, be reduced by lengthening the follow-up period for forward studies to increase the experience in terms of person-years observed. The larger sample size required for the forward study reflects principally the infrequent occurrence of the disease entity under investigation. In the example illustrated, uncovering 100 cases of disease in a forward study would require either 100,000 individuals with the factor or 1,000,000 without. For diseases with a higher probability of occurrence the disparity in required size between retrospective and forward studies would be progressively reduced.

The retrospective study might be looked upon as a natural extension of the practice of physicians since the time of Hippocrates, to take case histories as an aid to diagnosis. Its guise has varied with respect to the means of measuring the prevalence of the suspect factor among diseased persons and the criteria for determining unusual departures from normal experience. When an association is so marked, as in Percival Pott's observations on the representation of chimney sweeps among cases of scrotal cancer, no further quantitative data are required to perceive its significance.

The retrospective approach has often been employed in studies of communicable diseases, one illustration being Snow's observations (*1*) on a common water supply for cholera cases in an area served by several sources (there would have been no element of unusualness had there been but one water supply).   When a disease is epidemic in a circumscribed locality, the disease-free population in the same area offers a natural contrast.   The method may be used successfully for endemic diseases as well.   Holmes, in reaching his conclusions on the communicable nature of puerperal fever (*2*), noted particularly that a large number of women with puerperal fever had been attended by the same physicians.   In this context it should be emphasized that communicable disease investigations have often combined retrospective and forward study methods.   For example, Snow supplemented his retrospective observations on water supply by a contrast of cholera rates among subscribers of the Southwark and Vauxhall water company with the experience of persons served by the Lambeth water company within the same area.

When a disease occurs sporadically, or its occurrence is not confined to a well-defined group (such as women at childbirth), a choice of controls is not immediately evident.   For cancer and other diseases characterized by high fatality rates, a study restricted to decedents might use persons dying from other causes as controls.   Rigoni Stern adopted this technique in deducing the relationship of cancer of the breast and of the uterus to pregnancy history (*3*).   Some contemporary studies have also used deaths from other causes as controls (*4*, *5*).

The present-day controlled retrospective studies of cancer date from the Lane-Claypon paper on breast cancer published in 1926 (*6*).   This report is significant in setting forth procedures for selecting matched hospital controls and relating them to a consideration of study objectives. Retrospective techniques have since been applied in several investigations of cancer, including the following partial list of current references for a few primary sites: bladder (*7–10*), breast (*11–13*), cervix (*13–16*), larynx (*17, 18*), leukemia (*19*), lung (*18, 20–27*), and stomach (*13, 28–30*).

Statisticians have been somewhat reluctant to discuss the analysis of data gathered by retrospective techniques, possibly because their training emphasizes the importance of defining a universe and specifying rules for counting events or drawing samples possessing certain properties. To them, proceeding from "effect to cause," with its consequent lack of specificity of a study population at risk, seems an unnatural approach. Certainly, the retrospective study raises some questions concerning the representative nature of the cases and controls in a given situation which cannot be completely satisfied by internal examination of any single set of data.

Only a few published papers have treated the statistical aspects of retrospective studies.   Cornfield discussed the problem in terms of estimated measures of relative and absolute risks arising from contrasts of persons with and without specified characteristics (*31*).   His paper was concerned with the simple situation of a homogeneous population of cases and controls, presumably alike in all characteristics except the one under investigation, which could be represented by a single contingency table. In a later contribution he handled the problem of controlling for other variables by adjusting the distribution of controls to the observed distribution of cases (16). Dorn briefly mentions retrospective studies with emphasis on such topics as sources of data, choice of controls, and validity of inferences (32).

This paper presents a method for computing relative risks for retrospective study contrasts, which controls for the effects of other variables by use of the basic statistical principle of subclassification of data. The related problem of significance testing is also considered. Since details of statistical treatment are conditioned by study objectives, data collection methods, choice of a control series, and the use of matched or unmatched controls, these topics are also discussed briefly.

Objectives

Retrospective studies are relatively inexpensive and can play a valuable role as scouting forays to uncover leads on hitherto unknown effects, which can then be explored further by other techniques. The effects may be novel and not suggested by existing data, as in the pioneer work on the association of smoking and lung cancer or the association of blood type and gastric cancer, or they may represent refinements of current knowledge. The latter category might include collection of lifetime residence and/or work histories to elaborate differences in incidence and mortality which appear when some diseases are classified by last place of residence or last occupation of the newly diagnosed case or decedent.

With diseases of low incidence the controlled retrospective study may be the only feasible approach. Here emphasis should be placed on assembling results from several studies. Before accepting a finding and offering an interpretation, scientific caution calls for ascertaining whether it can be reproduced by others and in other administrative settings having their own peculiar biases.

A primary goal is to reach the same conclusions in a retrospective study as would have been obtained from a forward study, if one had been done. Even when observations for a forward study have been collected, a supplementary retrospective approach to the same body of material may prove useful in collecting more data on points not covered in the original study design or in amplifying suggestive associations appearing in the initial forward-study results.

The findings of a retrospective study are necessarily in the form of statements about associations between diseases and factors, rather than about cause and effect relationships. This is due to the inability of the retrospective study to distinguish among the possible forms of association—cause and effect, association due to common causes, etc. Similar difficulties of interpretation arise in forward studies as well. A forward study, to avoid these difficulties, would need to be performed with the preciseness of a laboratory experiment. For example, such a study of associations with cigarette smoking would require that an investigator randomly assign his subjects in advance to the various smoking categories, rather than simply note the categories to which they belong. The inherent practical difficulties of such an enterprise are evident.

In addition to the failings shared with the forward study, the retrospective study is further exposed to misleading associations arising from the circumstances under which test and control subjects are obtained. The retrospective study picks up factors associated with becoming a diseased or a disease-free *subject*, rather than simply factors associated with presence or absence of the disease. The difficulties in this regard may be most pronounced when the study group represents a cross section of patients alive at any time (prevalence), including some who have been ill for a long period. Inclusion of the latter may lead to identification of items associated with the course of the illness, unrelated to increased or decreased risk of developing the disease. The theoretical point has been raised that factors conducive to longer survival of patients may be found in "prevalence" samples and interpreted erroneously as being associated with excess liability to the disease (*33*). Loopholes of this type are minimized when investigations are restricted to samples of newly diagnosed patients (incidence).

A partial remedy for these uncertainties lies in employing a conservative approach to interpretation of the associations observed. Recognizing the ease with which associations may be influenced by extraneous factors, the investigator may require not only that the measure of relative risk be significantly different from unity but also that it be importantly different. He may, for instance, require that the data indicate an increased relative risk for a characteristic of at least 50 percent, on the assumption that an excess of this magnitude would not arise from extraneous factors alone. However, the use of such conservative procedures emphasizes a corresponding need to pinpoint the disease entity under study. A strong relationship between a factor and a disease entity might fail to be revealed, if the entity was included in a larger, less well-defined, disease category. After the event from data now at hand, we know that a study of the association of cigarette smoking with epidermoid and undifferentiated pulmonary carcinoma is more revealing than an inquiry covering all histologic types of lung cancer.

Multiple Comparison Problem

The present-day retrospective study is usually concerned with investigating a variety of associations with a disease, little effort being involved in acquiring, within limits, added information from respondents. The results may be analyzed in a number of ways: the various factors may be investigated separately, without regard to the other factors; they may be investigated in conjunction with each other, a particular conjunction being considered a factor in its own right; or, more commonly, a factor may be tested with control for the presence or absence of other factors. Thus, if the role of cigarette smoking and coffee drinking in a given disease are under study, the possible comparisons include the relative risk of disease for individuals who both smoke and drink as opposed to all other persons, or as opposed to those who neither smoke, nor drink coffee. In addition, the relative risk associated with smoking might be obtained separately for drinkers and nondrinkers of coffee, with a weighted average of these two relative risks constituting still another item. Conversely, risks associated with coffee drinking, with adjustments for cigarette smoking, could be computed.

The potential comparisons arising from a comprehensive retrospective study can be large. Almost any reasonable level of statistical significance used to test a single contrast, when applied to a long series of contrasts, will, with a high degree of probability, result in some contrasts testing significant, even in the absence of any real associations. The usual prescription for coping with this multiple comparison problem—requiring individual comparisons to test significant at an extreme probability level to reduce the number of associations incorrectly asserted to be true— would result only in making real associations difficult to detect.

However, the multiple comparison problem exists only when inferences are to be drawn from a single set of data. If the purpose of the retrospective study is to uncover leads for fuller investigation, it becomes clear there is no real multiple significance testing problem—a single retrospective study does not yield conclusions, only leads. Also, the problem does not exist when several retrospective and other type studies are at hand, since the inferences will be based on a collation of evidence, the degree of agreement and reproducibility among studies, and their consistency with other types of available evidence, and not on the findings of a single study.

Nevertheless, it would be wise to employ testing procedures which do not lead to a superabundance of potential clues from any one study. This may be achieved by employing nominal significance levels in testing factors of primary interest incorporated into the design of an investigation and applying more stringent significance tests to comparisons of secondary interest or to comparisons suggested by the data. For the usual problem of multiple significance testing, this would be equivalent to allocating a large part of the desired risk of erroneous acceptance of an association as real to a small group of comparisons where fruitful results were anticipated, and parceling out the remainder of the available risk to the large bulk of comparisons of a more secondary nature. This minimizes the risk of diluting, through inclusion of many secondary comparisons, the chances for detecting an important primary effect.

Representative Nature of Data

The fundamental assumption underlying the analysis of retrospective data is that the assembled cases and controls are representative of the universe defined for investigation. This obligates the investigator· not only to examine the data which are the end product but also to go behind the scenes and evaluate the forces which have channeled the material to his attention, including such items as local practices of referral to specialists and hospitals and the patient's condition and the effect of these items on the probability of diagnosis or hospital admission. We re-emphasize that this requires the exercise of judgment on the potential magnitude of biases and as to whether they could result in factors seeming to be related to a disease, in the absence of a real association of the factor with presence or absence of the disease. The danger of bias may be greatest in working with material from a single diagnostic source or institution.

Among the more important practical considerations affecting retrospective studies is that they are ordinarily designed to follow the line of least resistance in obtaining case and control histories. This means that cases and controls will often be hospital patients rather than persons in the general population outside hospitals. As a result, any factor which increases the probability that a diseased individual will be hospitalized for the disease may mistakenly be found to be associated with the disease. For example, Berkson (*34*) and White (*35*) have pointed out that positive association between two diseases, not present in the general population, may be produced when hospital admissions alone are studied, because persons with a combination of complaints are more likely to require hospital treatment. In theory, bias might also be produced in reverse manner, if the suspect factor diminished the probability of hospitalization for other diagnoses used as controls. The difficulties are not unique for hospital patients. Similar loopholes in interpretation may be advanced for any special groups used as sources of cases and controls.

However, a mere catalogue of biases arising from the possibly unrepresentative nature of a sample of cases and controls should not *ipso facto* invalidate any study findings. This is a substantive issue to be resolved on its merits for a specific investigation. Collateral evidence may provide information on the potential magnitude of bias and the size of spurious associations which could result. In some situations the difference between cases and controls may be so great that postulation of an unreasonably large bias would be required. Whether he consciously recognizes it or not, the investigator must always balance the risks confronting him and decide whether it is more important to detect an effect, when present, or to reject findings, when they may not reflect the true situation. If opportunities for further testing exist, one should not be too hasty in rejecting an association as an artifact arising from the method of data collection, and in foreclosing exploration of a potentially fruitful lead.

Because of the important role retrospective studies play in studies of human genetics, mention may be made of a bias frequently encountered in studies dealing with the familial distribution of diseases. A frequently used procedure takes a group of diagnosed cases for a disease in question and a group of controls and compares the prevalence of this disease among relatives of the probands and controls. The bias arises from the unrepresentative nature of the probands with respect to familial distribution and is known in other fields as "the problem of the index case" or "the effect of method of ascertainment." It has long been recognized that the characteristics for a random sample of families will differ from those for families to whom the investigator's attention has been directed because the family rosters include individuals selected for study on the basis of a specified attribute. For example, data on family size (number of children) obtained from siblings, rather than parents, are biased, since two or three potential index cases are present in the population for two- and three-child families as opposed to one for one-child families and none for childless couples. The analogy for disease occurrence is apparent. Families with two or three cases of the disease under study may have double or triple the probability of being represented by individuals in source material and having a representative selected as a proband than families with only one case. An appropriate analysis for this situation in studies of family size and birth order has been discussed by Greenwood and Yule (*36*), which takes account of the probability of family representation in proband data. Haenszel (*37*) has applied their correction to gastric-cancer data reported by Videbaek and Mosbech (*38*) and found the correction to reduce the originally reported fourfold excess of gastric cancer among relatives of probands, as compared to relatives of controls, to one of about 60 percent.

One remedy for the weakness of the retrospective approach to problems involving association of diseases and familial distribution would be to place greater reliance on forward observations of defined cohorts for data on these topics.

Controls

While easier accessibility to and lesser expense of hospital controls are important considerations, they should not deter one from collecting control data for a sample representing a more general population, if the latter are demonstrably superior. Some of the uncertainties about the superiority of hospital or general population controls arise from the need to maintain comparability in responses. The dependence of retrospective studies on comparability of responses from cases and controls cannot be overemphasized. When more accurate answers can be obtained from controls in a medical-care environment, the gain in comparability of responses for these controls could outweigh the other advantages to be derived from the more representative nature of general population controls. The difficulties may be illustrated by the experience with smoking histories. Hospital controls invariably yield a higher proportion of smokers for each sex than controls of comparable age drawn from the general population (*27*). Does this mean more complete smoking histories are collected in hospitals or does it imply that smokers have higher hospital admission rates? If the first alternative is correct, hospital controls are the appropriate choice for measuring the association of smoking history with a given disease. The second alternative calls for general population controls and in this situation the use of hospital controls yields underestimates of the degree of association.

Dual hospital and general population controls would have some merit. If control data from the two sources were in agreement, this would rule out some alternative interpretations of the findings. In the event of disagreement, its extent could be measured and alternate calculations made on the degree of association between an event and a suspect antecedent characteristic. Where the two sets of controls lead to substantially different results, a cautious and conservative interpretation is indicated.

Some topics, such as those bearing on sex practices and use of alcohol, may be amenable to study only within a clinical setting, and the collection of general population data on these items may prove impractical. The limitations of general population controls in this regard may have been overstressed, and empirical trials to test what information can be collected in household surveys should be encouraged instead of dismissing the possibility with no investigation whatsoever. Whelpton and Freedman, for example, have reported some success in collecting histories of contraceptive practices in interviews of a random sample of housewives (39).

When hospital controls are chosen, some precautions may be built into the study. Within limitations on the nature of controls imposed by a study hypothesis, controls drawn from a wide variety of diseases or admission diagnoses should be preferred. This permits examination of the distribution of the study characteristics among subgroups to check on internal consistency or variation among controls. This affords protection against two sources of error: a) attributing an association to the disease under investigation, when the effect is really linked to the diagnosis from which controls were drawn, and b) failure to detect an effect because both the study and control diseases are associated with the suspect factor. The latter is far from impossible. Both tuberculosis and bronchitis have exhibited association with smoking history and the use of one disease or the other as a control could easily lead to missing the association with smoking history. Similarly, patients with coronary artery disease would not constitute suitable controls for a study of the relationship of smoking and bladder cancer and *vice versa*, since the investigator would probably conclude that smoking was not related to either disease, when in truth it appears related to both. When there is definite evidence that two diseases are associated, for example, pernicious anemia and stomach cancer, the use of one as a control for the other is contraindicated, unless the study is specially designed to elucidate some aspects of the relationship.

It is always advantageous to include several items in a questionnaire for which general population data are available. This could be considered a partial substitute for dual hospital and general population controls. Disparity among cases, hospital controls, and general population controls on several general characteristics unrelated to the study hypothesis may be regarded as warning signals of the unrepresentative nature of the hospital cases and controls.

Where possible, interviews should be conducted without knowledge of the identity of cases and controls to guard against interviewer bias, although administrative reasons will often prevent attainment of "blind" interviews. In cooperative studies employing several interviewers, the magnitude of interviewer bias may be diminished, since it is unlikely that all interviewers will share the same bias in concert. In special circumstances, such as those prevailing at Roswell Park Memorial Institute, admissions may be interviewed before diagnosis, and hence before the identity of cases and controls is established. This feature requires a comprehensive, general purpose interview routinely administered to all admissions, which may restrict its use to publicly supported institutions diagnosing and treating neoplastic diseases or other specialized disease entities. Several epidemiological contributions for specific cancer sites have been based on the unique control data available from Roswell Park Memorial Institute (9, 11, 12, 30, 40–43), which are particularly valuable for collation with studies depending on more conventional sources of controls to evaluate interviewer bias and related issues.

Some patients interviewed as diagnosed cases will subsequently have their diagnoses changed. This may be turned to advantage. If scrutiny of the data for the erroneously diagnosed group reveals they had histories resembling those for the control rather than the case series, as Doll and Hill found in their study of smoking and lung cancer (21), this would constitute evidence against interviewer bias.

In investigations of a cancer site the association of a factor may often be restricted to a specific histologic type or a well-defined portion of an organ. The finding that epidermoid and undifferentiated pulmonary carcinoma is more strongly related to smoking history than adenocarcinoma of the lung is now well established. The range of explanations for the observed deficit of epidermoid carcinoma of the cervix in Jewish women as compared to other white women is greatly circumscribed by the presence of about equal numbers of adenocarcinoma of the corpus in both groups. When these finer diagnostic details or their significance are unknown to the interviewer, another check on interviewer bias is provided. Furthermore, the confirmation in repeated studies of an association limited to a specific histologic type or a detailed site will lend credence to an etiological interpretation of the association. Repeated confirmation is an essential element. Otherwise, a very specific association may be a reflection of the multiple comparison problem; if enough contrasts are created by fractionation of a single set of data, some apparently significant result is likely to appear. For this reason it would be desirable to reproduce such provocative results as Wynder's finding that use of alcohol was more strongly associated with cancer of the extrinsic larynx than of the intrinsic larynx (18), and Billington's report that prepyloric and cardiac neoplasms of the stomach were associated with blood group A and those located in the fundus with blood group O (44).

Discussion of matched controls in relation to the analysis and the computation of relative risks is deferred to a later section. One consideration on matched controls arising in the planning and development of a study should be mentioned here. Obviously, if the risk of disease changes with age an apparent association of the disease with other age-related factors may result. Other apparent associations with race, sex, nativity, etc., may arise in a similar manner. In devising rules for selecting controls, those factors known or strongly suspected to be related to disease occurrence should be taken into account if unbiased and more precise tests of the significance of the factors under investigation are desired. A sensible rule is to match those factors, such as age and sex, the effect of which may be conceded in advance and for which strong evidence is available from other sources, such as mortality data and morbidity surveys. When a factor is matched, however, it is eliminated as an independent study variable; it can be used only as a control on other factors. This suggests caution in the amount of matching attempted. If the effect of a factor is in doubt, the preferable strategy will be not to match but to control it in the statistical analysis. While the logical absurdity of attempting to measure an effect for a factor controlled by matching must be obvious, it is surprising how often investigators must be restrained from attempting this.

When a minimum of matching is involved, the importance of establishing, precisely and in advance, the method by which controls are selected for study increases. The rule should be rigid and unambiguous to avoid creating effects by subconscious selection and manipulation of controls. The problem is similar to that encountered in therapeutic trials where a protocol spelling out all the contingencies and actions to be taken in advance is, along with random assignment of cases and controls, the major bulwark against bias.

To reduce interview time and expense there are advantages in procedures for selecting controls which permit a case and the corresponding controls to be interviewed in a single session, particularly if travel to several institutions is involved. In practice, this favors selecting controls from a hospital patient census rather than from hospital admission lists. The difficulty with hospital admissions is that there is no guarantee that the controls will be available in the hospital at the time the diagnosed case is interviewed. This point seems more important than the fact that patients with diagnoses requiring long-term stays are overrepresented in a current hospital census (45). If the latter is an important issue, it may be handled in analysis through subclassification of controls by diagnosis.

Normally there will be little difficulty in reconciling these considerations into a harmonious set of rules. The items to be matched often lend themselves to a procedure for specifying controls. In a recent study on female lung cancer we found that the definition of two controls as the next older and the next younger women in the same hospital service, present on the day the case was interviewed, met the requirements just outlined (27). The controls were uniquely defined, the records establishing their identity were readily available on the service floor, interviews could be completed in one day, and a provision for balancing ages of cases and controls was incorporated. Simultaneous interviews of cases and controls may be more than an administrative convenience. If the prevalence of the associated factor is rapidly shifting over time, failure to control time of interview could obscure or exaggerate an association.

Some Statistical Tools

To progress further, questions on the representative nature of the case and control series must have been resolved affirmatively. With this condition in mind, let us suppose that a controlled retrospective study has been conducted and that the number of diseased cases, N_1, consists of A individuals with the factor being investigated and B free of the factor, while the number of controls, N_2, consists of C individuals with, and D individuals without the factor. Let $M_1 = A + C$, $M_2 = B + D$, $T = N_1 + N_2 = M_1 + M_2 = A + B + C + D$. What statistical evidence is there for the presence of an association and what is an appropriate measure of the strength of the association?

A commonly employed statistical test of association is the chi-square test on the difference between the cases and controls in the proportion of individuals having the factor under test. A corrected chi square may be calculated routinely as

$$(|AD - BC| - \tfrac{1}{2}T)^2 T / N_1 M_1 N_2 M_2$$

and tested as a chi square with 1 degree of freedom in the usual manner.

A suggested measure of the strength of the association of the disease with the factor is the apparent risk of the disease for those with the factor, relative to the risk for those without the factor. Consider that a population falls into the four possible categories and in the proportions indicated by the following table:

	With factor	Free of factor	Total
With disease	P_1	P_2	$P_1 + P_2$
Free of disease	P_3	P_4	$P_3 + P_4$
Total	$P_1 + P_3$	$P_2 + P_4$	1

The proportion of persons with the factor having the disease is $P_1/(P_1 + P_3)$, while the corresponding proportion for those free of the factor is $P_2/(P_2 + P_4)$. Relatively then, the risk of the disease for those with the factor is $P_1(P_2 + P_4)/P_2(P_1 + P_3)$. On a sampling basis this quantity may be estimated either by drawing a sample of the general population and estimating P_1, P_2, P_3, and P_4 therefrom or estimating $P_1/(P_1 + P_3)$ and $P_2/(P_2 + P_4)$ separately from samples of persons with, and persons free of, the factor.

It may be noted, however, that if the relative risk as defined equals unity, then the quantity P_1P_4/P_2P_3 will also equal unity. Further, for diseases of low incidence where the values for P_1 and P_2 are small in comparison with P_3 and P_4 it follows, as has been pointed out by Cornfield (31), that P_1P_4/P_2P_3 is also a close approximation to the relative risk. This latter approximate relative risk can properly be estimated from the two sample approaches described or from samples drawn on a retrospective basis; that is, separate samples of persons with, and persons free of, the disease. The sample proportions of persons with, and free of, the factor in the retrospective approach provide estimates of $P_1/(P_1 + P_2)$ and of $P_2/(P_1 + P_2)$ from the sample having the disease and of $P_3/(P_3 + P_4)$ and of $P_4/(P_3 + P_4)$ from the disease-free sample. The estimate of P_1P_4/P_2P_3 is obtained by appropriate multiplication and division of these four quantities.

Whichever of the three methods of sampling is employed, the estimate of the approximate relative risk, P_1P_4/P_2P_3, reduces simply to AD/BC, where A, B, C, and D are defined in the manner stated in the first paragraph of this section. Also, the chi-square test of association given, which is essentially a test of whether or not the relative risk is unity, is equally applicable to all three sampling methods.

In the foregoing the two basic statistical tools of the epidemiologist for retrospective studies, the chi-square significance test and the measure of a relative risk, have been described for a relatively simple situation, one in which to all intents there is a single homogeneous population. The more complex situations confronting the epidemiologist in actual practice and the corresponding modifications in the statistical procedures will be presented.

Two other statistical problems may be noted here. One is the determination of how large a retrospective study to conduct. This depends on how sure we wish to be that the study will yield clear evidence that the relative risk is not unity, when it in fact differs from unity to some important degree. Application of this statistical technique requires reinterpreting a relative risk greater than unity into the corresponding difference between the diseased and the disease-free groups in the proportion of persons with the factor. For example, suppose an attack rate of 20 percent, given a normal rate of 10 percent, is worth uncovering. Suppose further that the factor associated with the increased disease rate affects 20 percent of the population. The population would then be distributed as follows:

	With factor	Free of factor	Total
With disease	$P_1 = 4\%$	$P_2 = 8\%$	12%
Free of disease	$P_3 = 16\%$	$P_4 = 72\%$	88%
Total	20%	80%	100%

The required retrospective study should be large enough to differentiate between a 33.3 percent $[P_1/(P_1 + P_2)]$ relative frequency of the factor among diseased individuals and an 18.2 percent $[P_3/(P_3+P_4)]$ relative frequency among disease-free individuals. The usual procedures for determining required sample sizes to differentiate between two binomial proportions are applicable in this situation.

While rigorous extension of this procedure to the more complex situations to be considered is not too simple, it can readily be adapted to secure approximations of the necessary study size. One might, for example, start by estimating the over-all required sample size following the procedure just indicated for differentiating between two sample proportions, assuming that cases and controls are homogeneous with respect to factors other than the one under investigation. Suppose on an over-all basis it is determined that the study should include $N_1 = 200$ disease cases and $N_2 = 200$ controls, but that the study data will be sub-classified for purposes of analysis. Ignoring mathematical complications resulting from variations in binomial parameter values within individual subclassifications, we may interpret the above values of N_1 and N_2 as roughly meaning that the total information required for the study is $N_1 N_2/(N_1 + N_2) = 100$. The objective should then be to assign values to N_{1i} and N_{2i} to obtain a total score of 100 for the cumulated information over all the subclassifications, $\Sigma N_{1i} N_{2i}/(N_{1i} + N_{2i})$, where N_{1i} and N_{2i} are the number of cases and controls in the ith subclassification.

This formulation of required total information brings out some aspects of retrospective study planning which are considered later in this paper. For instance, if any N_{1i} or N_{2i} is zero, no information is available from that particular category. Much of the benefit of a large N_{1i} (or N_{2i}) in any particular category is lost if the corresponding N_{2i} (or N_{1i}) is small. It is normally desirable to have N_{1i} and N_{2i} values commensurate with each other; for fixed totals, ΣN_{1i} and ΣN_{2i}, the total information in an investigation will be at a maximum if the degree of crossmatching is equal in all subclassifications with a constant case-control ratio of $\Sigma N_{1i}/\Sigma N_{2i}$. Maintaining a fixed case-control ratio among categories need not preclude assigning more cases and controls to specific categories. Larger numbers may be desired for categories of crucial interest to the study or for categories which represent greater segments of the population.

The information formula also reveals the limits for adjusting the relative numbers of diseased and control cases. It shows that if the number of controls (N_2) becomes indefinitely large, the required N_1 value can at most be reduced only by a factor of 2. Furthermore, this reduction in required diseased cases may be inappropriate if one wishes to obtain clear results for the separate subcategories.

The study size requirements suggested by the information formula may be seriously in error if the binomial parameters show excessive variation among subcategories. Ordinary precautions, however, should serve to keep the formula useful. In some situations it may be desirable to modify the information formula indicated above to reflect the contribution due to variation in the binomial parameters involved.

The second statistical procedure involves setting reasonable limits on the relative risk when it is in fact different from unity. For the homogeneous case considered, formulas for such limits have been published in (46). The chi-square test as stated is essentially a test of whether or not the confidence limits include unity. Extension of this procedure to more complex cases is fairly involved and depends primarily on the measure of relative risk adopted. In the absence of a clear justification for any single measure of over-all relative risk, the burden of extremely involved computation of confidence limits in such cases would not seem warranted. Instead, we feel that emphasis should be directed to obtaining an over-all measure of risk, coupled with an over-all test of statistical significance.

Statistical Procedures for Factor Control

A major problem in any epidemiological study is the avoidance of spurious associations. It has been remarked that where the risk of disease changes with age, apparent association of the disease with other age-related factors can result. However, there are appropriate statistical procedures for controlling those factors known or suspected to be related to disease occurrence. They serve not only to remove bias from the investigation but, in addition, can add to its precision.

Two simple procedures for obtaining factor control may first be mentioned. One is simply to restrict the investigation to individuals homogeneous on the factors to be controlled. For this situation the statistical procedures already outlined would be appropriate. The potential number of individuals available for such a study would, of course, be sharply restricted.

There is also the matching case method. A sample of N diseased individuals is drawn and the characteristics of each individual noted with respect to the control factors. Subsequently, a sample of N well individuals is drawn, with each individual matched on the control factors to one of the diseased individuals. The statistical procedures to be presented can be shown to cover the matched-sample approach as a special case, and a discussion of the analysis of such data will be given in that context. Some difficulties of the matched-sample study may be mentioned here. One is that when matching is made on a large number of factors, not even the fiction of a random sampling of control individuals can be maintained. Instead, one must be grateful for each matching control available. Another difficulty is that the method cannot be applied to factors under control, since diseased and control individuals are identical with respect to these factors. Conversely, factors under study in matched samples cannot themselves be controlled statistically. They can be analyzed separately or in particular conjunctions but cannot be employed as control factors.

An alternative to case matching is to draw independent samples of cases and controls, and adjust for other factors in the analysis. This approach requires simply the classification of individuals according to the various control and study factors desired, and an analysis for each separate subclassification as well as an appropriate summary analysis. Its success will depend on a reasonable degree of cross-matching between observations on diseased and control persons. In a small study various devices for reducing the number of subclassifications and for increasing the chances of cross-matching may be necessary, including a limit on the number of factors on which individuals are classified in any one analysis and the use of broad categories for any particular classification. Thus, a 10-year interval for age classification might permit a reasonable degree of cross-matching, whereas a 1-month interval would not.

The need for some degree of deliberate matching, even when the classification approach is employed, can be seen. If the disease under consideration occurs at advanced ages, little cross-matching would result if controls were selected from the general population. The remedy lies in deliberately selecting controls from the same age groups anticipated for persons with the disease, perhaps even matching one or more controls on age for each diseased person. This principle can be extended to matching on several control factors, *solely for the purpose of increasing the extent of cross-matching in the analysis.*

One of the subtle effects which can occur in a retrospective study, even with careful planning, may be pointed out. It can be shown, for instance, that within a given age interval the average age of individuals with cancer of certain sites will be greater than the average age of individuals from the general population in the same age interval. This can arise when incidence increases rapidly with age and may pose a serious problem with broad age intervals. This effect can be offset by close matching of cases and controls on age in drawing samples, even though they are classified by a broad age category in the analysis.

When a random sample of diseased and disease-free individuals is classified according to various control factors the distribution of the factor under study within the *ith* classification may be represented as follows:

	With factor	Free of factor	Total
With disease	A_i	B_i	N_{1i}
Free of disease	C_i	D_i	N_{2i}
Total	M_{1i}	M_{2i}	T_i

Within this subgroup the approximate relative risk associated with the disease may be written as A_iD_i/B_iC_i. One may compare the observed number of diseased persons having the factor, A_i, with its expectation under the hypothesis of a relative risk of unity, $E(A_i)=N_{1i}M_{1i}/T_i$. The discrepancy between A_i and $E(A_i)$ (which is also the discrepancy for any other cell within a 2×2 table) can be tested relative to its variance which, subject to the fixed marginal totals—N_{1i}, N_{2i}, M_{1i}, and M_{2i}—is given by $V(A_i) = N_{1i}N_{2i}M_{1i}M_{2i}/T_i^2(T_i-1)$. The corrected chi square with 1 degree of freedom $(|A_i-E(A_i)|-\frac{1}{2})^2/V(A_i)$ reduces in this case to $(|A_iD_i-B_iC_i|-\frac{1}{2}T_i)^2(T_i-1)/N_{1i}N_{2i}M_{1i}M_{2i}$. This formula for the variance of A_i is obtained as the variance of the binomial variable $N_1PQ(P=M_1/T$, $Q = M_2/T)$, multiplied by a finite population correction factor $(T-N_1)/(T-1) = N_2/(T-1)$. The earlier chi-square formula, which is ordinarily used, essentially employs a finite population correction factor of N_2/T.

There is thus a difference between the two chi-square formulas of a factor of $(T-1)/T$ which, though trivial for any single significance test with respectably large T, can become important in the over-all significance test. It is with the latter formula, just presented, that chi square is computed as the ratio of the square of a deviation from its expected value to its variance.

The adjustment for control factors is at this point resolved for the resulting separate subclassifications. The problem of over-all measures of relative risk and statistical significance still remains. A reasonable over-all significance test which has power for alternative hypotheses, where there is a consistent association in the same direction over the various sub-classifications between the disease and a study factor, is provided by relating the summation of the discrepancy between observation and expectation to its variance. The corrected chi square with 1 degree of freedom then becomes $(|\Sigma A_i - \Sigma E(A_i)| - \frac{1}{2})^2 / \Sigma V(A_i)$ where $E(A_i)$ and $V(A_i)$ are defined as above.

The specification of a summary estimate of the relative risk associated with a factor is not so readily resolved as that for an over-all significance test, and involves consideration of alternate approaches to a weighted average of the approximate relative risks for each subclassification $(A_i D_i / B_i C_i)$. If one could assume that the increased relative risk associated with a factor was constant over all subclassifications, the estimation problem would reduce to weighting the several subclassification estimates according to their respective precisions. The complex maximum likelihood iterative procedure necessary for obtaining such a weighted estimate would seem to be unjustified, since the assumption of a constant relative risk can be discarded as usually untenable.

Another possible criterion for obtaining a summary estimate of relative risk would involve weighting the risks for subclassification by "importance." A twofold increase of a large risk is more important than a twofold increase of a small risk. An increased risk for a large group is more important than one for a small group. An increased risk for young individuals may be more important than for older individuals with a shorter life expectation. Difficulties arise in attempts to weight relative risk by measures of importance. For one, the necessary information on importance, in terms of the size of the populations affected or in terms of the absolute level of rates prevailing in the subgroups, is generally not contained within the scope of the investigation. A problem in definition of the precise terms of the weighted comparison also appears. Does one want to adjust the risks of disease among persons with the factor to the distribution of the population without the factor, or *vice versa*, or adjust the risks for the populations with and without the factor to a combined standard population? These procedures, and the different phrasing of the comparisons which they entail, could yield different answers. If only a small proportion of the population with the factor was in a subcategory with a high relative risk, while most of the factor-free population fell into this subcategory, and in other categories the relative risk associated with the factor was less than unity, the factor would appear to exert a protective influence under one set of weights but a harmful effect under the other.

Published instances of summary relative risks do not fall clearly into either of the two categories—weighting by precision or weighting by importance. They do follow an approach usually employed in age-adjusting mortality data. Since the relative risk for a single 2×2 table can be obtained from the incidence of the factor among diseased and well individuals, the problem would appear translatable into terms of obtaining over-all, category-adjusted incidence figures. Direct or indirect methods of adjustment can be used, employing as a standard of reference the frequency distribution or rates corresponding to the sample of diseased persons, of controls, or the diseased persons and controls combined.

While such adjustment procedures provide weighting by importance in their customary application to mortality rates, this is not so in the relative risk situation. This may be illustrated in the following extreme example. Suppose that in each of two subcategories the approximate relative risk for a contrast between the presence and absence of a factor is about 5, which arises in the first subcategory from contrasting percentages of 1 and 5, and in the second subcategory from contrasting percentages of 95 and 99. If these percentages were based on equal numbers of individuals, all methods of category adjusting would yield contrasting adjusted summary percentages of 46 and 52, and a resultant relative risk of slightly less than 1.3. Some other approach for obtaining category-adjusted relative risks would seem desirable. However, to the extent that such extreme situations are not encountered in actual practice, results based on these more conventional adjustment procedures will not be grossly in error.

A suggested compromise formula for over-all relative risk is given by $R = \Sigma(A_i D_i/T_i)/\Sigma(B_i C_i/T_i)$. As a weighted average of relative risks this formula would, in the illustration given, yield the over-all relative risk of 5 found in each of the two subcategories. The weights are of the order $N_{1i} N_{2i}/(N_{1i} + N_{2i})$ and as such can be considered to weight approximately according to the precision of the relative risks for each subcategory. The weights can also be regarded as providing a reasonable weighting by importance.

An interesting property of this summary relative risk formula is that it equals unity only when $\Sigma A_i = \Sigma E(A_i)$ and hence the corresponding chi square is zero. From the fact that $A_i - E(A_i) = (A_i D_i - B_i C_i)/T_i$, it follows that when $\Sigma A_i = \Sigma E(A_i)$, $\Sigma A_i D_i/T_i$ will equal $\Sigma B_i C_i/T_i$, chi square will be zero, and R will be unity. The chi-square significance test can thus be construed as a significance test of the departure of R from unity.

Of some other procedures for measuring over-all relative risks, the one following also has the interesting property of being equal to unity when $\Sigma(A_i) = \Sigma E(A_i)$ and therefore subject to the chi-square test:

$$R_1 = \frac{\Sigma A_i \Sigma D_i}{\Sigma B_i \Sigma C_i} \bigg/ \frac{\Sigma E(A_i) \Sigma E(D_i)}{\Sigma E(B_i) \Sigma E(C_i)} \text{ where } E(A_i) = N_{1i} M_{1i}/T_i, \ E(B_i)$$

$$= N_{1i} M_{2i}/T_i, \ E(C_i) = N_{2i} M_{1i}/T_i, \text{ and } E(D_i) = N_{2i} M_{2i}/T_i.$$

In this formula the numerator represents the crude value for the relative risk, which would result from pooling the data into one table and ignoring all subclassification on other factors. The denominator represents the crude value for relative risk, which would have resulted from pooling in the situation where all relative risks within each subclassification were exactly unity. Readers familiar with the "indirect" method of computing standardized mortality ratios will recognize an analogy between the "indirect" method and the above procedure.

The estimator R_1 can be seen to have a bias toward unity. One reason is covered by the illustration which indicated that adjusted percentages (or frequencies) do not yield an appropriate adjusted relative risk. In addition, when either cases or controls have little representation in a subcategory, there will be lack of cross-matching and little information about relative risk, and the observed cell frequencies and their expectations will be numerically close. Such results will, in the process of summation used by the estimator, tend to force its value toward unity. This weakness will not be too important if the degree of cross-matching is roughly equal in the various subclassifications—an optimum goal one would normally attempt to achieve. The bias will become more pronounced as the number of control factors increases and as the prospects for good cross-matching become poorer.

We used the estimator R_1 in a recent paper (27), knowing its potential weaknesses. This was done to present results more nearly comparable with those reported by other investigators using similarly biased estimators. One set of results from this paper on lung cancer among women illustrates the conservative behavior of estimator R_1 compared with R, as additional factors are controlled. The relative risk (R_1) for epidermoid and undifferentiated pulmonary carcinoma associated with smoking more than one pack of cigarettes daily as compared to nonsmokers decreased from 7.1 (controlled for age) to 5.6 (controlled for age and coffee consumption). The corresponding figures, with R as a measure of relative risk, were 9.7 and 9.9.

Computational procedures for R and R_1 are presented in table 1, drawing on material comparing smoking histories of women diagnosed as cases of epidermoid and undifferentiated pulmonary carcinoma with those of female controls. For simplicity in presentation only two smoking levels are considered—nonsmokers and smokers of more than one pack of cigarettes daily. An extension of the significance testing procedures to the case of study factors at more than two levels is discussed later. The control factors are age and occupation. The basic data are given in the first 9 columns. Columns 10 and 11 carry the derivative calculations required for R. Columns 12 and 13 are used in the computation for R_1 and for the variance estimate in column 14—the latter being needed for the chi-square test. Only columns 1 to 10, 12, and 14 would be necessary to compute chi square, R and R_1. Column 13 is not essential for the computation of $E(D)$ but simplifies computation of $V(A)$, while providing a check on $E(A)$. Column 11 serves as a check on 10 and 12. A system of checks and computations is outlined at the bottom of table 1. Not all the computations shown would ordinarily be necessary for an analysis.

The corrected chi-square value of 30.66 (1 degree of freedom) would indicate a highly significant association between epidermoid and undifferentiated pulmonary carcinoma and cigarette smoking in women, after adjusting for possible effects connected with age or occupation. The

738   MANTEL AND HAENSZEL

TABLE 1.—*Illustrative computations for chi square and for summary measures of undifferentiated pulmonary carcinoma*

Group	Epidermoid-undifferentiated pulmonary carcinoma			Controls			Cases and controls		
	1 + Pack cigarettes daily	Nonsmokers	Total	1 + Pack cigarettes daily	Nonsmokers	Total	1 + Pack cigarettes daily	Nonsmokers	Total
	A (1)	B (2)	N_1 (3)	C (4)	D (5)	N_2 (6)	M_1 (7)	M_2 (8)	T (9)
Housewives — under age 45	0	2	2	0	7	7	0	9	9
45–54	2	5	7	1	24	25	3	29	32
55–64	3	6	9	0	49	49	3	55	58
65 and over	0	11	11	0	42	42	0	53	53
White-collar workers — under age 45	3	0	3	2	6	8	5	6	11
45–54	2	2	4	2	18	20	4	20	24
55–64	2	4	6	2	23	25	4	27	31
65 and over	0	6	6	1	11	12	1	17	18
Other occupations — under age 45	1	0	1	3	10	13	4	10	14
45–54	4	1	5	1	12	13	5	13	18
55–64	0	6	6	1	19	20	1	25	26
65 and over	1	3	4	0	15	15	1	18	19
Total	18	46	64	13	236	249	31	282	313

Checks: Total discrepancy, Y, $= \Sigma A - \Sigma E(A) = \Sigma(1) - \Sigma(12) = 11.625$
$\quad\quad\quad = \Sigma D - \Sigma E(D) = \Sigma(5) - \Sigma(13) = 11.625$
$\quad\quad\quad = \Sigma(AD/T) - \Sigma(BC/T) = \Sigma(10) - \Sigma(11) = 11.625$
$\Sigma(15) + \Sigma(16) = 64.000; \ \Sigma(3) = 64$
$\Sigma(17) + \Sigma(18) = 249.000; \ \Sigma(6) = 249$
Derivative computations: $\Sigma E(B) = \Sigma(2) + Y = 57.625$
$\quad\quad\quad\quad\quad\quad \Sigma E(C) = \Sigma(4) + Y = 24.625$
$\quad\quad\quad\quad\quad\quad \Sigma(AT/N_1) = \Sigma(1) + \Sigma(17) = 94.960$
$\quad\quad\quad\quad\quad\quad \Sigma(BT/N_1) = \Sigma(2) + \Sigma(18) = 218.040$
$\quad\quad\quad\quad\quad\quad \Sigma(CT/N_2) = \Sigma(4) + \Sigma(15) = 16.325$
$\quad\quad\quad\quad\quad\quad \Sigma(DT/N_2) = \Sigma(5) + \Sigma(16) = 296.675$

value of R implies that the risk of these cancers is 10.7 times as great for women currently smoking in excess of 1 pack a day than for women who never used cigarettes. The value of R_1, 7.05, is almost identical with the crude relative risk, 7.10, which results from pooling the data with no attention to the control factors. The difference from the published R_1 value of 6.3 in (27) arises from the exclusion in the illustrative example, of data for women currently smoking 1 pack a day or less and for occasional or discontinued smokers.

The computation of three other summary estimates of relative risk is also outlined in table 1. The additional derivative computations required for this purpose appear in columns 15 to 18. All three estimates are based on a direct method of category adjustment, that is, the use of a standard distribution to which both the case and control distributions are *relative risk (R, R₁, R₂, R₃, and R₄) relating to the association of epidermoid and in women with smoking history*

			Derivative computations					
$\dfrac{AD}{T}$ $\dfrac{(1)(5)}{(9)}$	$\dfrac{BC}{T}$ $\dfrac{(2)(4)}{(9)}$	E(A) $\dfrac{(3)(7)}{(9)}$	E(D) $\dfrac{(6)(8)}{(9)}$	V(A) $\dfrac{(12)(13)}{(9)-1.0}$	$\dfrac{N_1C}{N_2}$ $\dfrac{(3)(4)}{(6)}$	$\dfrac{N_1D}{N_2}$ $\dfrac{(3)(5)}{(6)}$	$\dfrac{N_2A}{N_1}$ $\dfrac{(1)(6)}{(3)}$	$\dfrac{N_2B}{N_1}$ $\dfrac{(2)(6)}{(3)}$
(10)	(11)	(12)	(13)	(14)	(15)	(16)	(17)	(18)
0	0	0	7. 000	0	0	2. 000	0	7. 000
1. 500	0. 156	0. 656	22. 656	0. 480	0. 280	6. 720	7. 143	17. 857
2. 534	0	0. 466	46. 466	0. 380	0	9. 000	16. 333	32. 667
0	0	0	42. 000	0	0	11. 000	0	42. 000
1. 636	0	1. 364	4. 364	0. 595	0. 750	2. 250	8. 000	0
1. 500	0. 167	0. 667	16. 667	0. 483	0. 400	3. 600	10. 000	10. 000
1. 484	0. 258	0. 774	21. 774	0. 562	0. 480	5. 520	8. 333	16. 667
0	0. 333	0. 333	11. 333	0. 222	0. 500	5. 500	0	12. 000
0. 714	0	0. 286	9. 286	0. 204	0. 231	. 769	13. 000	0
2. 667	0. 056	1. 389	9. 389	0. 767	0. 385	4. 615	10. 400	2. 600
0	0. 231	0. 231	19. 231	0. 178	0. 300	5. 700	0	20. 000
0. 790	0	0. 211	14. 211	0. 166	0	4. 000	3. 750	11. 250
12. 825	1. 201	6. 375	224. 375	4. 036	3. 325	60. 675	76. 960	172. 040

Chi-square: $X^2 = (|\text{discrepancy}| - 0.5)^2/\Sigma V(A) = (|Y| - 0.5)^2/\Sigma(14) = 30.66$
Relative risk: $R = \Sigma(AD/T)/\Sigma(BC/T) = \Sigma(10)/\Sigma(11) = 10.68$
$R_1 \begin{cases} \text{crude relative risk, } f = \Sigma A\Sigma D/\Sigma B\Sigma C = \Sigma(1)\Sigma(5)/\Sigma(2)\Sigma(4) = 7.10 \\ \text{adjustment factor, } f = \Sigma E(A)\Sigma E(D)/\Sigma E(B)\Sigma E(C) = \Sigma(12\Sigma(13)/\Sigma E(B)\Sigma E(C) \\ \phantom{\text{adjustment factor, } f} = 1.0081 \\ R_1 = r/f = 7.05 \end{cases}$
$R_2 = \Sigma A\Sigma(N_1D/N_2)/\Sigma B\Sigma(N_1C/N_2) = \Sigma(1)\Sigma(16)/\Sigma(2)\Sigma(15) = 7.14$
$R_3 = \Sigma(N_2A/N_1)\Sigma D/\Sigma(N_2B/N_1)\Sigma C = \Sigma(5)\Sigma(17)/\Sigma(4)\Sigma(18) = 8.12$
$R_4 = \Sigma(AT/N_1)\Sigma(DT/N_2)/\Sigma(BT/N_1)\Sigma(CT/N_2) = 7.91$

Note: Figures shown are rounded from those actually calculated and consequently are not fully consistent. Column totals and figures shown do not necessarily agree.

adjusted. If the distribution of diseased cases is taken as the standard distribution to which the controls are adjusted, the estimator becomes

$$R_2 = \frac{\Sigma A_i \Sigma\left(D_i \times \dfrac{N_{1i}}{N_{2i}}\right)}{\Sigma B_i \Sigma\left(C_i \times \dfrac{N_{1i}}{N_{2i}}\right)}.$$

Estimator R_2 was used by Wynder *et al.* in a study of the association of cervical cancer in women with circumcision status of sex partners *(16)*. The merit of employing the cervical cancer case-distribution as the standard presumably rests on the fact that this distribution at least would be well defined by the study.

If the distribution of control cases is taken as standard the estimator becomes

$$R_3 = \frac{\Sigma \left(A_i \times \dfrac{N_{2i}}{N_{1i}} \right) \Sigma D_i}{\Sigma \left(B_i \times \dfrac{N_{2i}}{N_{1i}} \right) \Sigma C_i}.$$

If the combined distribution is taken as standard the estimator becomes

$$R_4 = \frac{\Sigma \left(A_i \times \dfrac{T_i}{N_{1i}} \right) \Sigma \left(D_i \times \dfrac{T_i}{N_{2i}} \right)}{\Sigma \left(B_i \times \dfrac{T_i}{N_{1i}} \right) \Sigma \left(C_i \times \dfrac{T_i}{N_{2i}} \right)}.$$

If any N_{1i} or N_{2i} should equal zero, the estimator R_4 would not be defined. R_2 is not defined for any zero-valued N_{2i}, and R_3 is not defined for any zero-valued N_{1i}. In these instances it would be necessary to exclude the zero-frequency categories to define the estimators. The estimator R_1 retains these categories at the expense of greater bias toward unity. The estimator R gives such categories zero weight, since they contain no information about relative risk. The chi-square significance test gives no weight to these categories.

While R_4 is clearly a direct adjusted estimate of relative risk employing the combined distribution as standard, R_2 and R_3 may be viewed alternatively as either direct or indirect adjusted estimates. The same estimates will result if a direct adjustment is made using the distribution of cases as standard, or an indirect adjustment is made using the factor incidence rates for controls as the standard rates.

It may be noted that in the example used, the values for R_2, R_3, and R_4 (7.14, 8.12, and 7.91, respectively) were roughly comparable to R_1, and all were smaller than R. The example was selected because all the N_{1i} and N_{2i} values were non-zero, so that the values of R_2, R_3, and R_4 were all defined.

The over-all relative risk estimates are averages and as averages may conceal substantial variation in the magnitudes of the relative risk among subgroups. Ordinarily, the individual subcategory data should be examined, paying special attention to relative risks based on reasonably large sample sizes. This will provide protection against the potential deficiencies of any particular summary relative risk formula employed. The over-all chi-square significance test in any case will remain appropriate for detecting any strong general tendency for the risk of disease to be associated with the presence or absence of the test factor.

The Matched-Sample Study

The matched-sample study previously described can be considered a special case of the classification procedure with the number of classifications equal to the number of pairs of individuals. The status of pairs of well and diseased individuals classified with respect to the presence or absence of the suspect factor in each individual will be represented as

F, G, H, or J in the following fourfold table. The meanings attached to the marginal totals A, B, C, and D are the same as those in the first schematic representation.

Well individuals	Diseased individuals		
	With factor	Free of factor	Total
With factor	F	G	C
Free of factor	H	J	D
Total	A	B	N

In the absence of association between the disease and the factor, we expect the same number of individuals with the factor to appear among both diseased and well individuals; that is, we expect $A(=F + H)$ to equal $C(=F + G)$. This can occur only when $G = H$ and the statistical test is simply whether or not G differs significantly from 50 percent of $G + H$. G is tested as a binomial variable with parameter $\frac{1}{2}$, $G + H$ being the number of cases. G thus has expectation $\frac{1}{2}(G + H)$, variance $\frac{1}{4}(G + H)$ and the corrected chi square with 1 degree of freedom can readily be shown to reduce to $(|G - H| - 1)^2/(G + H)$.

Treating the data as consisting of N classifications each with $N_{1i} = N_{2i} = 1$, $T_i = 2$ and applying the previously described procedures will lead to the same value of chi square. For F of the N classifications, $A_i = 1$, $M_{1i} = 2$, $M_{2i} = 0$, $E(A_i) = 1$, $V(A_i) = 0$; for G classifications $A_i = 0$, $M_{1i} = M_{2i} = 1$, $E(A_i) = \frac{1}{2}$, $V(A_i) = \frac{1}{4}$; for H classifications $A_i = 1$, $M_{1i} = M_{2i} = 1$, $E(A_i) = \frac{1}{2}$, $V(A_i) = \frac{1}{4}$; and for J classifications, $A_i = 0$, $M_{1i} = 0$, $M_{2i} = 2$, $E(A_i) = 0$, $V(A_i) = 0$. Thus, $\Sigma A_i = F + H$, $\Sigma E(A_i) = F + \frac{1}{2}(G + H)$, $\Sigma V(A_i) = \frac{1}{4}(G + H)$, and the resultant corrected chi square can again be seen to be $(|G - H| - 1)^2/(G + H)$.

It is of interest to observe that the summary chi-square formula is appropriate in the matched-sample case, even though the frequencies for each of the separate subclassifications are small. Its appropriateness, despite the small frequencies, stems from the fact that it is a test on a summation of random variables, A_i, and thus tends to approach normality rapidly, making the chi-square test valid, even though the individual A_i's are not normally distributed. This property of the chi-square formula applies in the general classification as well as the matched-sample situation. Only substantial lack of cross-matching in the general case would tend to make the chi-square test invalid. It is also essential, of course, that there be some appreciable variation in the presence or absence of the factor under study.

It should be noted that in the matched-sample study with $T_i = 2$ for each of the N pairs of individuals, the variances of the A_i's would have been understated by a factor of 2, had $T - 1$ been replaced by T in the variance formulas. The usual formula for chi square does essentially make this replacement, but it is usually of little consequence if T is of any reasonable magnitude. The formulas for relative risk in the matched-sample study reduce simply to the following: $R = H/G$; $R_1 = R_2 = R_3 = R_4 = AD/BC$.

Study Factors at More Than Two Levels

The preceding discussion on the analysis or retrospective data has been in terms of the test factor under study taking only two values. This framework has sufficed for discussion of the underlying statistical ideas and issues. In practice, the study factor will frequently take on more than two, perhaps many, potential values. When the number of study factor values is large, grouping can reduce them to manageable proportions.

The need to consider only a limited number of classes for the study factor stems from the fact that, when an association is anticipated, most of the significant information about the association will come from the results for the more extreme values of the study factor. While it is efficient to concentrate attention on the test factor classes expected to show the greatest differences in association with the disease, it is also profitable to consider intermediate values for the test factor to seek evidence for a consistent pattern of association. For example, in table 1, a highly significant difference between nonsmokers and women currently smoking more than 1 pack of cigarettes daily was illustrated. Inclusion of data for smokers of 1 pack or less a day showing results intermediate between the other classes would have added little, if anything, to the statistical significance of the results, and might actually lower it, if one made an over-all test of the differences among the three smoking classes. However, the observation that the intermediate smoking class does, in fact, show an intermediate relative risk contributes to an orderly pattern and increases our confidence in the conclusions suggested by the data for the remaining two classes.

For any two particular test-factor levels, the relative risk for one over the other may be calculated using only the data pertaining to those two levels or by using the results for all test levels. In the formulas previously given for R, R_1, R_2, R_3, and R_4, the difference between the two calculating procedures is simply one of setting the values of N_{1i}, N_{2i}, and $T_i = N_{1i} + N_{2i}$ in terms of number of cases and controls occurring at the two study-factor levels only, or defining them in terms of total number of cases and controls in the entire study. When total cases and controls are used in defining N_{1i}, N_{2i}, and T_i, it can be shown that for R_1, R_2, R_3, and R_4 the various relative risks will be internally consistent with each other. If the relative risk for the first level is twice that for the second level, which in turn is twice that for the third level, then the relative risk for the first level will be four times that of the third. These exact relationships do not hold for R as an estimator of relative risk, and a somewhat sophisticated extension of the formula for R would be required to secure this property.

The problem of obtaining a summary chi square when the study factor is at more than two levels is complicated by the fact that the deviations from expectation at the various study-factor levels are intercorrelated. When there are but two levels, the two deviations will have perfect negative correlation, and attention need be directed to only one of the deviations.   Irrespective of the number of levels, at any one level the deviation from expectation among diseased persons will be equal, but opposite in sign, to the deviation from expectation among controls, so that attention can be confined to the deviations for diseased persons.

The prob'.m can be stated as one of reducing a set of correlated deviations into a summary chi square.   Table 2 applies this process for obtaining a summary chi square to the study of the association of epidermoid and undifferentiated pulmonary carcinoma in women and maximum cigarette-smoking rate, classified into three levels, after adjustment for age and occupation.

The general expressions for the expectations and variances of the number of cases at a particular test-factor level are given in the lower right section of table 2.   Also shown is the expression for the covariance between the number of cases at two different test-factor levels.   Since the total of all the deviations is zero, one would in general need the variances of, and covariances between, the number of cases at all but one of the levels.   The number of covariance terms will rise sharply as the number of test levels are increased.   At 3 test levels, there are 2 variance terms and 1 covariance term, while at 10 test levels, there. would be 9 variances and 36 covariance terms of interest.

For the general case the burden of computation could be heavy.   After all the necessary computation for the deviations, their variances and covariances, there would still remain the problem of converting these, presumably by matrix methods, into a summary chi square.   Since the retrospective problem will normally involve only a limited number of test-fact^r levels, precise procedures will be given only for the three-level situation, and approximate procedures outlined for the general case.

The exact computation procedure for the three-level case is detailed in table 2.   Lines (1), (2), and (4) show the total observed and expected frequencies and variances of the number of cases (and controls) at each of the three smoking-rate levels, after adjusting for age and occupation.   These are the summary totals over each subclassification obtained by application of the formulas appearing in table 2.

Lines (5) and (6) give the chi squares corresponding to the total deviation from expectation at each of the smoking-rate levels.   The chi squares in line (5) are corrected for continuity.   They relate to the difference of the particular level to which they apply, from the two other levels combined.   Following the usual practice of making no continuity corrections when chi squares with more than 1 degree of freedom are under consideration, line (6) shows the uncorrected chi squares.

The computing procedure of table 2 takes advantage of the fact that, since the sum of the deviations from expectation is zero, the variance of the third deviation must equal the sum of the other two variances plus twice the covariance for the first two deviations.   The covariance of the first two deviations is readily obtained as illustrated and is used in calculating the summary chi square.   The summary chi square is obtained as the sum of squares of two orthogonal deviates, with each

TABLE 2.—*Illustrative computation of summary chi square, when there are 3 levels for study factor. The data relate to the association of epidermoid and undifferentiated pulmonary carcinoma in women with smoking history*

	1 + Pack cigarettes daily			1 Pack or less of cigarettes daily			Occasional or nonsmokers			Total		
	Epidermoid-undifferentiated pulmonary carcinoma	Controls	Total (ΣM_1)	Epidermoid-undifferentiated pulmonary carcinoma	Controls	Total (ΣM_2)	Epidermoid-undifferentiated pulmonary carcinoma	Controls	Total (ΣM_3)	Epidermoid-undifferentiated pulmonary carcinoma (ΣN_1)	Controls (ΣN_2)	Total (ΣT)
(1) Total observed frequencies	19	17	36	32	71	103	51	251	302	102	339	441
(2) Total expected frequencies, adjusted for age and occupation	9.09	26.91	36	23.76	79.24	103	69.15	232.85	302	102	339	441
(3) Total deviation from expectation (1) − (2)	$+9.91 = Y_1$			$+8.24 = Y_2$			$-18.15 = Y_3$					
(4) Variance of total observed frequencies, subject to fixed marginal totals in each age and occupation group	$5.9163 = V_1$			$12.2900 = V_2$			$14.0723 = V_3$					
(5) Individual corrected chi squares $(\lvert Y\rvert-0.5)^2/V$	$14.97 = X_{1c}^2$			$4.88 = X_{2c}^2$			$22.15 = X_{3c}^2$					
(6) Individual uncorrected chi squares Y^2/V	$16.60 = X_1^2$			$5.53 = X_2^2$			$23.42 = X_3^2$					

(7) Covariance (Y_1, Y_2) $(V_3 - V_1 - V_2)/2$ .... -2.0670

(8) Adjusted Y_2, $Y_3 - (7)Y_1/V_1$ 11.70

(9) Adjusted V_2, $V_3 - (7)^2/V_1$ 11.5678

(10) Adjusted X_2^2, $(8)^2/(9)$ .... $11.83 = X_2^2(\text{ad.})$

(11) Summary chi square (2 degrees of freedom) $X_1^2 + X_2^2(\text{ad.})$ .... $16.60 + 11.83 = 28.43$

For the general situation the total expected case frequency at the jth level of a test factor is

$$\sum_i N_{1i} M_{ji}/T_i$$

The variance of the total case frequency is

$$V_j = \sum_i \frac{N_{1i} N_{2i} M_{ji}(T_i - M_{ji})}{T_i^2(T_i-1)}$$

The covariance of the total case frequencies at test levels j and k is

$$-\sum_i \frac{N_{1i} N_{2i} M_{ji} M_{ki}}{T_i^2(T_i-1)}$$

The index of summation, i, represents the various subclassifications into which the results are divided

For 3 test levels only, since $Y_3 = -(Y_1 + Y_2)$, it follows that $V_3 = V_1 + V_2 + 2$ Covariance (Y_1, Y_2)

square adjusted for its own variance. The first deviate squared is simply the uncorrected chi square at the first level in line (6)—the variance of the deviate remaining as initially calculated. The second deviate is the deviation at the second level adjusted for its correlation with the first deviation [adjusted $Y_2 = Y_2 - b_{21}Y_1$; $b_{21} =$ covariance (Y_1, Y_2)/variance Y_1)]. The variance of the adjusted second deviate is the initial value reduced by that portion of the variation accounted for by the first deviation [Var. (adjusted Y_2) = variance $Y_2 -$ covariance$^2(Y_1, Y_2)$/variance Y_1)].

In the present instance the summary chi square with 2 degrees of freedom is 28.43 [line (11)]. This presumably is close to the chi square with 1 degree of freedom which would have obtained had only the two most extreme smoking classes been compared. If one examines the individual uncorrected chi squares [line (6)], their total is found to be 45.55, the maximum individual figure being 23.42. *It will necessarily be true that the summary chi-square value will lie between the largest of the three chi squares and their total. At almost any reasonable probability level these limits would be sufficient to establish statistical significance without further calculation.* In our companion paper (27) this rule sufficed in almost all instances to separate the significant from the nonsignificant results.

Comments on Extensions to More Than Three Factors

Two procedures can be suggested for getting approximate summary chi squares, when there are a large number of levels for the test factors, without the burden of computation that the exact method would entail. Both methods calculate the approximate summary chi square as a sum of squares of approximately orthogonal standardized deviates.

In the first method one computes an uncorrected chi square with 1 degree of freedom for the difference of the first level from all the remaining levels combined (the same first step as in the illustration for the three-level case). Discarding the data from the first level, a second chi square is computed for the difference between the second test-factor level and the remaining levels combined. This is done successively up to and including the last two remaining levels. The approximate summary chi square is then the sum of the separate chi squares with the number of degrees of freedom being one less than the number of test levels.

Exactly orthogonal standardized deviates would be obtained if, in the summary analysis, as each successive total deviation from expectation were evaluated, it was adjusted for its multiple regression on the preceding deviations, and then standardized by the adjusted variance. This, of course, would no longer be a simplified approximate procedure. However, it can be shown that for a single classification, in the multiple regression of any deviation from expectation on any subset of deviations, the regression coefficients will all be equal; the multiple regression on the set of deviations will be the same as the simple regression on their sum. The equality of regression coefficients, while holding true exactly for deviations in the separate subclassifications, will hold only approximately for the total deviations from expectation (it would hold exactly if equal numbers of individuals were observed from level to level at each subclassification). Nevertheless, this result suggests that approximately orthogonal deviates would be obtained if, in evaluating each successive total deviation, it were adjusted for the cumulative total of deviations already evaluated. Computing procedures to accomplish this can readily be devised.

Both approximate chi-square procedures just outlined, which may have merit when more than three groups are being compared simultaneously, should, in theory, yield linear combinations of independent chi squares. While testing the chi-square values obtained as though they were exact is not likely to be too inappropriate, it may be more correct to obtain a modified number of degrees of freedom, along the lines suggested by Satterthwaite (47) for problems involving such linear combinations. What the modified number of degrees of freedom would be has not been investigated by us, and it may prove as easy to apply the exact chi-square procedure, indicated later, as to determine the appropriate degrees of freedom for the approximate chi square.

It is of interest that a somewhat similar task of obtaining an appropriate summary chi square appears in the birth-order problems described by Halperin (48). There, it was necessary to compare a set of total observations (across family sizes) with a set of total expectations, one for each birth order. Halperin described a matrix-inversion procedure for reducing the set of correlated deviations into a summary chi square. In that problem it can be shown that all the regression coefficients are equal in the multiple regression of the deviation at a particular birth order on the set of deviations at all succeeding birth orders. The second approximate method described previously for the present problem could thus be used exactly for the birth-order problem, permitting simplified computation of chi square. The procedure indicated by Halperin has the advantage of generality and could be applied to the current and related problems, if one obtained all the necessary variances and covariances and inverted the resulting matrix.

References

(1) SNOW, J.: On the mode of communication of cholera. *In* Snow on Cholera. New York, The Commonwealth Fund, 1936, pp. 1–139.

(2) HOLMES, O. W.: The contagiousness of puerperal fever. *In* Medical Classics. Baltimore, Williams & Wilkins Co., vol. 1, 1936, pp. 211–243.

(3) STERN, R.: Nota sulle ricerche del dottore Tanchon intorno la frequenza del cancro. Annali Universali di Medicina 110: 484–503, 1844.

(4) STOCKS, P., and CAMPBELL, J. M.: Lung cancer death rates among non-smokers and pipe and cigarette smokers. Brit. M. J. 2: 923–929, 1955.

(5) WYNDER, E. L., and CORNFIELD, J.: Cancer of the lung in physicians. New England J. Med. 248: 441–444, 1953.

(6) LANE-CLAYPON, J. E.: A further report on cancer of the breast, with special reference to its associated antecedent conditions. Rept. Publ. Health & M. Subj., No. 32, 1926, pp. 1–189.

(7) CLEMMESEN, J., LOCKWOOD, K., and NIELSEN, A.: Smoking habits of patients with papilloma of urinary bladder. Danish M. Bull. 5: 123–128, 1958.

(8) DENOIX, P. R., and SCHWARTZ, D.: Tobacco and cancer of the bladder. (Bulletin de L'Association francaise pour l'étude du Cancer.) Cancer 43: 387–393, 1956.

(9) LILIENFELD, A. M., LEVIN, M. L., and MOORE, G. E.: The association of smoking with cancer of the urinary bladder in humans. A.M.A. Arch. Int. Med., 1956.

(10) MUSTACCHI, P., and SHIMKIN, M. B.: Cancer of the bladder and infestation with *Schistosoma hematobium.* J. Nat. Cancer Inst. 20: 825–842, 1958.

(11) LILIENFELD, A. M.: The relationship of cancer of the female breast to artificial menopause and marital status. Cancer 9: 927–934, 1956.

(12) LILIENFELD, A. M., and LEVIN, M. L.: Some factors involved in the incidence of breast cancer. *In* Proc. Third National Cancer Conference. Philadelphia, J. B. Lippincott Co., 1957, pp. 105–112.

(13) SEGI, M., FUKUSHIMA, I., FUJISAKU, S., KURIHARA, M., SAITO S., ASANO, K., and KAMOI, M.: An epidemiological study on cancer in Japan. Gann Supp. 48, 1957.

(14) DUNHAM, L. J., THOMAS, L. B., EDGCOMB, J. H., and STEWART, H. L.: Some environmental factors and the development of uterine cancers in Israel and New York City. To be published in Acta Unio internat. contra cancrum.

(15) STOCKS, P.: Cancer of the uterine cervix and social conditions. Brit. J. Cancer 9: 487–494, 1955.

(16) WYNDER, E. L., CORNFIELD, J., SCHROFF, P. D., and DORAISWAMI, K. R.: A study of environmental factors in carcinoma of the cervix. Am. J. Obst. & Gynec. 68: 1016–1052, 1954.

(17) MILLS, C. A., and PORTER, M. M.: Tobacco smoking habits and cancer of the mouth and respiratory system. Cancer Res. 10: 539–542, 1950.

(18) WYNDER, E. L., BROSS, I. J., and DAY, E.: A study of environmental factors in cancer of the larynx. Cancer 9: 86–110, 1956.

(19) MANNING, M. D., and CARROLL, B. E.: Some epidemiological aspects of leukemia in children. J. Nat. Cancer Inst. 19: 1087–1094, 1957.

(20) BRESLOW, L., HOAGLIN, L., RASMUSSEN, G., and ABRAMS, H. K.: Occupations and cigarette smoking as factors in lung cancer. Am. J. Pub. Health 44: 171–181, 1954.

(21) DOLL, R., and HILL, A. B.: A study of the aetiology of carcinoma of the lung. Brit. M. J. 2: 1271–1286, 1952.

(22) LEVIN, M. L.: Etiology of lung cancer; present status. New York J. Med. 54: 769–777, 1954.

(23) SADOWSKY, D. A., GILLIAM, A. G., and CORNFIELD, J.: The statistical association between smoking and carcinoma of the lung. J. Nat. Cancer Inst. 13: 1237–1258, 1953.

(24) WATSON, W. L., and CONTE, A. J.: Lung cancer and smoking. Am. J. Surg. 89: 447–456, 1955.

(25) WYNDER, E. L., and GRAHAM, E. A.: Tobacco smoking as possible etiologic factor in bronchiogenic carcinoma. J.A.M.A. 143: 329–336, 1950.

(26) WYNDER, E. L., BROSS, I. J., CORNFIELD, J., and O'DONNELL, W. E.: Lung cancer in women. New England J. Med. 255: 1111–1121, 1956.

(27) HAENSZEL, W., SHIMKIN, M. B., and MANTEL, N.: A retrospective study of lung cancer in women. J. Nat. Cancer Inst. 21: 825–842, 1958.

(28) AIRD, I., BENTALL, H. H., and ROBERTS, J. A. F.: A relationship between cancer of stomach and the ABO blood groups. Brit. M. J. 1: 799–801, 1953.

(29) BUCKWALTER, J. A., WOHLWEND, C. B., COLTER, D. C., TIDRICK, R. T., and KNOWLER, L. A.: The association of the ABO blood groups to gastric carcinoma. Surg. Gynec. & Obst. 104: 176–179, 1957.

(30) KRAUS, A. S., LEVIN, M. L., and GERHARDT, P. R.: A study of occupational associations with gastric cancer. Am. J. Pub. Health 47: 961–970, 1957.

(31) CORNFIELD, J.: A method of estimating comparative rates from clinical data. Applications to cancer of the lung, breast, and cervix. J. Nat. Cancer Inst. 11: 1269–1275, 1951.

(32) DORN, H. F.: Some applications of biometry in the collection and evaluation of medical data. J. Chron. Dis. 1: 638–664, 1955.

748   MANTEL AND HAENSZEL

(33) NEYMAN, J.: Statistics—servants of all sciences. Science 122: 3166, 1955.

(34) BERKSON, J.: Limitations of the application of fourfo'd table analysis to hospital data. biometrics Bull. 2: 47–53, 1946.

(35) WHITE, C.: Sampling in medical research. Brit. M. J. 2: 1284–1288, 1953.

(36) GREENWOOD, M., and YULE, G. U.: On the determination of size of family and of the distribution of characters in order of birth from samples taken through members of the sibships. Roy. Stat. Soc. J. 77: 179–197, 1914.

(37) HAENSZEL, W.: Variation in incidence of and mortality from stomach cancer with particular reference to the United States. J. Nat. Cancer Inst. 21: 213–262, 1958.

(38) VIDEBAEK, A., and MOSBECH, J.: The aetiology of gastric carcinoma elucidated by a study of 302 pedigrees. Acta med. scandinav. 149: 137–159, 1954.

(39) WHELPTON, P. K., and FREEDMAN, R.: A study of the growth of American families. Am. J. Sociol. 61: 595–601, 1956.

(40) LEVIN, M. L., GOLDSTEIN, H., and GERHARDT, P. R.: Cancer and tobacco smoking. J.A.M.A. 143: 336–338, 1950.

(41) LEVIN, M. L., KRAUS, A. S., GOLDBERG, I. D., and GERHARDT, P. R.: Problems in the study of occupation and smoking in relation to lung cancer. Cancer 8: 932–936, 1955.

(42) LILIENFELD, A. M.: Possible existence of predisposing factors in the etiology of selected cancers of nonsexual sites in females. A preliminary inquiry. Cancer 9: 111–122, 1956.

(43) WINKELSTEIN, W., JR., STENCHEVER, M. A., and LILIENFELD, A. M.: Occurrence of pregnancy, abortion and artificial menopause among women with coronary artery disease: a preliminary study. J. Chron. Dis. 7: 273–286, 1958.

(44) BILLINGTON, B. P.: Gastric cancer—relationships between ABO blood-groups, site, and epidemiology. Lancet 2: 859–862, 1956.

(45) SCHWARTZ, D., and ANGUERA, G.: Une cause de biais dans certaines enquêtes médicales: le temps de séjour des malades a l'hôpital. Communication à l'Institut International de Statistique, 30ème Session. Stockholm, 1957.

(46) CORNFIELD, J.: A statistical problem arising from retrospective studies. Proc. Third Berkeley Symposium on Mathematical Statistics and Probability 4: 135–148, 1956.

(47) SATTERTHWAITE, F. E.: Synthesis of variance. Psychometrika 6: 309–316, 1941.

(48) HALPERIN, M.: The use of X^2 in testing effect of birth order. Ann. Eugenics 18: 99–106, 1953.

*U.S. GOVERNMENT PRINTING OFFICE: 1981-0-341-812/2023

II-6.

Olli S. Miettinen: Components of the Crude Risk Ratio. American Journal of Epidemiology 1972; 96:168–172.

Miettinen's "Components of the Crude Risk Ratio" could have equally as well appeared in Part I, as I think the most important contribution of this paper was in the realm of causal (as distinct from statistical) inference: the recognition of the standardized morbidity ratio (SMR) (and not some other adjusted risk ratio, such as Mantel-Haenszel) as the fundamental causal component of the crude risk ratio.

The idea of factorizing the crude risk ratio into two components, one due to confounding and one due to exposure effect, had been earlier employed by Bross [1966]. It was Miettinen, however, who recognized a general principle underlying such factorization. This principle is implicit in the paragraph following equation 1 of the paper. Miettinen stated that confounding could be estimated by "simulating the removal of the effect of exposure," that is, by estimating how many exposed cases would remain out of the total number of exposed cases, e, if the excess caseload attributable to exposure was removed from the case series. Estimation of the number of these "residual" cases, e^*, led immediately to the recognition of the "standardized morbidity ratio" e/e^* as the component of the crude ratio due to exposure effect. In the absence of other assumptions, this estimate of exposure effect was properly computed by treating all quantities except e, the total number of exposed cases, as fixed.

Miettinen's arguments were widely misunderstood, and despite Miettinen's warnings in his discussion (p. 171), e^* was often confused with the chi-square null expectation. The latter is computed by treating the total number of cases ($e + f$), rather than the number of unexposed cases (f), as fixed. At other times the component of the crude risk ratio due to confounding (equation 2 of the paper) was confused with the risk ratio for the confounder's effect on risk. Miettinen [1977] attempted to address the latter confusion, and elsewhere I have attempted to address the former [Greenland, 1986], but I suspect these distinctions are still not as widely appreciated as they should be.

A technical error occurs in the paper on page 169: here Miettinen states that for person-year denominators his SMR estimate, e/e^*, is the maximum-likelihood estimate (MLE) of a common relative risk, and that this is approximately so when the denominators are counts and the rates are low. This is in fact false in either case; the MLE has no closed form [Breslow 1984], and e/e^* approximates the MLE only if, in each stratum, the number of unexposed cases (f_j) is very large relative to the number of exposed cases (e_j) (with low rates needed as well if the denominators are counts). In general, e/e^* will have a larger variance than the MLE.

References:
Breslow NE. Elementary methods of cohort analysis. Int J Epidemiol 1984; 13:112–115.
Bross IDJ. Spurious effects from an extraneous variable. J Chron Dis 1966; 19:637–647.
Greenland S. Adjustment of risk ratios in case-base studies (hybrid epidemiologic designs). Statist Med 1986; 5:579–584.
Miettinen OS. The author replies. Am J Epidemiol 1977; 106:191–193.

AMERICAN JOURNAL OF EPIDEMIOLOGY
Copyright © 1972 by The Johns Hopkins University

Vol. 96, No. 2
Printed in U.S.A.

COMPONENTS OF THE CRUDE RISK RATIO

OLLI S. MIETTINEN[1]

(Received for publication December 17, 1971)

Miettinen, O. S. (Harvard School of Public Health, Boston, Mass. 02115). Components of the crude risk ratio. *Am J Epidemiol* 96: 168–172, 1972.—Both in cohort and case-control studies the estimate of the crude risk ratio factors into two important and easily derived components. One is a measure of the strength of confounding, and the other is an estimate of the residual risk ratio in terms of the standardized morbidity (mortality) ratio. For case-control studies the latter seems to be a new and useful "summary relative risk."

epidemiologic methods; biometry

Risk ratio ("relative risk" (RR)) is a parameter of central interest in epidemiology. It is defined as the ratio of the risk among the exposed to that among the nonexposed, with "risk" referring to some measure of morbidity or mortality and "exposure" and "nonexposure" distinguishing between a pair of alternative experiences or characteristics. The data-layouts for its estimation in cohort and case-control studies, respectively, are presented in table 1. With a cohort study the "crude" RR is estimated naturally by the ratio of the two observed rates, i.e., by $\hat{\rho}_c = (e/F)/(g/H) = eH/gF$. The equivalent formula for case-control studies, introduced by Cornfield (1), is the "odds ratio" $\hat{\rho}_c = ad/bc$ as long as the compared series are independent (unmatched) and the disease is "rare" among exposed as well as nonexposed individuals.

These estimates of the crude RR are useful for predictive purposes, but in etiologic research it is necessary to make a distinction between two components of the parameter—one resulting from recognizable confounding and the other possibly due to the effect of exposure. Customarily, analyses in such studies have been focused on the estimation of the latter component with no explicit assessment of the strength of confounding. However, the quantitation of confounding may contribute importantly even to the evaluation of the effect of exposure. For example, it may show that the control of certain factors is unnecessary in the analysis—a welcome finding in the face of the common problem of vanishing numbers when the subjects are stratified by several potentially confounding factors. Moreover, routine assessment of the amount of confounding in the crude RR would help accumulate valuable experience for use in the planning and evaluation of other studies.

The present paper describes methods of breaking the crude RR down to the two components. Secondarily, it may give some new insight into the interrelationship between cohort and case-control studies.

COHORT STUDIES

Suppose that the exposed and nonexposed series have been divided into strata of the confounding factor(s), and that in the jth stratum the data layout analogous to the one in table 1 has entries e_j, F_j, g_j and H_j. With $\sum e_j = e$, $\sum F_j = F$, $\sum g_j$ and g

Abbreviations: ML, maximum likelihood; RR, risk ratio; SMR, standard morbidity (mortality) ratio.

[1] Departments of Epidemiology and Biostatistics, Harvard School of Public Health, and Department of Cardiology, Children's Hospital Medical Center, Boston, Massachusetts.

Supported by grants 5 P01 CA 06373 and HE 10436 from the National Institutes of Health.

and $\sum H_j = H$ the estimate of the crude RR is, as before,

$$\hat{\rho}_c = eH/gF. \qquad (1)$$

The component attributable to confounding by the stratification factor(s) may be estimated by simulating the removal of the effect of the exposure within each stratum. This removal would have no bearing on the nonexposed series, and generally only a negligible effect, if any, on the distribution of exposed subjects among the strata. Thus, for considering this hypothetical case of no effect of the exposure we may keep the values of g_j, H_j and F_j unchanged. On the other hand, each e_j is replaced by the estimated "null" value of $e_j{}^* = g_j F_j/H_j$ corresponding to $\hat{\rho}_j = 1$. The estimate of the RR component, ρ^*, attributable to confounding by the stratification factors may then be taken as

$$\hat{\rho}^* = e^*H/gF, \qquad (2)$$

where $e^* = \sum e_j{}^*$.

The estimation of the residual RR, ρ_r, associated with the exposure conditionally on the stratification factors (i.e., with their effects removed) is a familiar problem. Among the exposed, a total of e events were observed as against an estimated "expected" number of e^* based on the rates in the nonexposed series, and the usual estimate of the residual RR is the standardized morbidity (mortality) ratio (SMR):

$$\hat{\rho}_s = e/e^*. \qquad (3)$$

Even though this ratio is the core element in "indirect standardization" with the nonexposed group as the "standard" (in the sense of stratum-specific rates), it should be regarded as the ratio of *"directly"* standardized rates for the exposed and nonexposed— i.e., an estimate of *standardized RR*—with the *exposed* group as the standard (in the sense of distribution over the strata). If the RR is the same for all the strata, and if the events are referred to person-years of follow-up (so that e_j and g_j can be regarded as realizations for independent Poisson variates), then e/e^* is the maximum likelihood

TABLE 1

Data-layouts in cohort and case-control studies, respectively

	Cohort study		Case-control study	
	Compared series			Compared series	
	Exposed	Nonexposed		Cases	Controls
Events*	e	g	Exposed	a	c
Denominator†	F	H	Nonexp.	b	d

* No. of cases of disease or death.

† No. of individuals studied or person-years of follow-up.

(ML) estimate of the common RR. With count denominators the above statistic is the ML estimate of a common RR only in the limit when the rates (of attack or prevalence) are very low, but it is a reasonable estimate even in less extreme situations.

It is apparent from the above formulas that the estimates of the components of RR are multiplicative, i.e., that

$$\hat{\rho}_c = \hat{\rho}^*\hat{\rho}_s. \qquad (4)$$

CASE-CONTROL STUDIES

In case-control studies with substantial numbers of subjects at each stratum an argument analogous to the one above can be used to estimate ρ^*, and the procedure suggests a simple estimate for ρ_s as well. Under the rare disease assumption the hypothetical removal of the effect of exposure induces no appreciable change in the control series nor in the distribution of nonexposed cases over the strata (even though the proportion of nonexposed individuals among all cases would change if the exposure in fact had an effect). For estimating ρ^* we may, therefore, keep the values of c_j, d_j and b_j unchanged, whereas each a_j is replaced by the "null" value of $a_j{}^* = b_j c_j/d_j$ which makes $\hat{\rho}_j = 1$. Thus the estimate becomes

$$\hat{\rho}^* = a^*d/bc, \qquad (5)$$

where $a^* = \sum a_j{}^*$.

170   OLLI S. MIETTINEN

TABLE 2

Drug-attributed rash in relation to allopurinol exposure among recipients of ampicillin. The Boston Collaborative Drug Surveillance Program (3)

Rash	Males Allopurinol			Females Allopurinol			Total Allopurinol		
	+	−	Total	+	−	Total	+	−	Total
+	5	36	41	10	58	68	15	94	109
−	33	645	678	19	518	537	52	1163	1215
Total	38	681	719	29	576	605	67	1257	1324
$\hat{\rho}$	2.49			3.42			2.99		

For estimating ρ_s we first observe that the jth stratum provides the estimate of $a_jd_j/b_jc_j = a_j/a_j^*$, the ratio of the observed number of exposed cases to the respective estimated expectation—analogously to e_j/e_j^* in the case of cohort studies. This analogy with cohort studies suggests that a reasonable overall estimate of the residual component in the large-sample case is

$$\hat{\rho}_s = a/a^*, \qquad (6)$$

which—like e/e^* in cohort studies—is the ratio of the observed total number of exposed cases to the estimate of its "expected" value under the assumption that $\rho_j \equiv 1$. Moreover, a/a^* must have the interpretation of being the sample value for the standardized RR, *with the exposed individuals in the source population as the standard* (in the sense of distribution over the strata). This inference can be directly verified: As noted above, the sample standardized RR is $\hat{\rho}_s = \sum w_j\hat{R}_{1j}/\sum w_j\hat{R}_{0j}$, where the w's are the weights of ("direct") standardization, and the $\hat{R}_1$'s and $\hat{R}_0$'s are rates in the exposed and nonexposed series, respectively. By definition, then, $\hat{\rho}_s = \sum w_j\hat{R}_{0j}\hat{\rho}_j/ \sum w_j\hat{R}_{0j}$. With the exposed individuals in the source population as the standard we may set w_j proportional to c_j/f_j, where f_j is the sampling fraction of noncases in the jth stratum. The values of $\hat{R}_{0j}$ may be taken proportional to $b_j/(d_j/f_j)$ as long as the

sampling fraction for cases is uniform over the strata. These substitutions, together with $\hat{\rho}_j = a_jd_j/b_jc_j$, yield

$$\hat{\rho}_s = \sum a_j/ \sum (b_jc_j/d_j) = a/a^*.$$

This proof also underscores the fact that the above interpretation of a/a^* as a standardized RR presupposes that the *cases be representative* of all cases in the source population, whereas the control series may be either representative of noncases or matched.

As with cohort studies, it is seen that $\hat{\rho}_c = \hat{\rho}^*\hat{\rho}_s$.

The above method of estimating the components of risk ratio should not be used in the small-sample case, particularly if d_j takes on small values. In the extreme, a single $d_j = 0$ can make $a^* = \infty$ and, consequently, $\hat{\rho}^* = \infty$ and $\hat{\rho}_s = 0$. When the values of c_j tend to be larger than those of d_j, a more stable measure of residual RR is obtained by using the *nonexposed as the standard* (in the sense of distribution over the strata) and computing

$$\hat{\rho}_s = b^*/b, \qquad (7)$$

where $b^* = \sum (a_jd_j/c_j)$. In the case of uniform RR over the strata a generally applicable, though computationally often somewhat cumbersome, approach is one where the ML estimate is first derived for $\hat{\rho}_r$, and $\hat{\rho}^*$ is then obtained from the relationship $\hat{\rho}^* = \hat{\rho}_c/\hat{\rho}_r$. A description of the ML estimation has been given recently by Gart (2).

EXAMPLES

Example 1. Table 2 presents some drug surveillance data analyzed in the spirit of *cohort* studies. Specifically, the frequency of drug-attributed rash is related to Allopurinol exposure among recipients of Ampicillin, and sex is treated as a potential confounding factor. The estimate of the crude risk ratio is $\hat{\rho}_c = 15(1257)/94(67) = 2.99$. Simulating the removal of the Appopurinol effect we have $e_1^* = 36(38)/681 = 2.01$ and $e_2^* = 58(29)/576 = 2.92$, and the risk ratio related to confounding by sex there-fore has the estimate $\hat{\rho}^* = (2.01 + 2.92)$ $(1257)/94(67) = 0.98$. This indicates that there is no material confounding by sex even though the rash rate has a rather strong relationship to sex among the nonex-posed, being $36/681 = 5.3$ per cent in males and $58/576 = 10.1$ per cent in females; the reason for the absence of confounding by sex is that the exposure rates in males and females are similar, namely $38/719 = 5.3$ per cent and $29/605 = 4.8$ per cent, respectively. The estimate of possibly Allo-purinol-attributable, standardized risk ratio is $\hat{\rho}_s = 15/(2.01 + 2.92) = 3.04$. The inter-relationship of $\hat{\rho}_c = \hat{\rho}^*\hat{\rho}_s$ is found to hold, as $2.99 = 0.98 (3.04)$ apart from round-off inaccuracy. If in this example there was a need to stratify by other factors, the lack of sex confounding would permit omission of stratification by sex.

Example 2. Table 3 gives data from a *case-control* study of the relationship of oral contraceptive use to venous thrombosis with age as a confounding factor. The esti-mate of the crude risk ratio is $\hat{\rho}_c = 12(347)/53(30) = 2.62$. The component of this at-tributable to confounding by age is not fully estimable from the data presented, inasmuch as there is residual age confound-ing within the 10-year categories considered. Ignoring this problem, we may compute $a_1^* = 39(18)/158 = 4.44$ and $a_2^* = 14(12)/189 = 0.89$, and these give as the estimate of the risk ratio component attributable to confounding by age in the 20–39-year range $\hat{\rho}^* = (4.44 + 0.89)(347)/53(30) = 1.16$. The estimate of the standardized com-ponent is $\hat{\rho}_s$ $12/(4.44 + 0.89) = 2.25$. The product of these two components is $1.16 (2.25) = 2.62$, the value of the crude risk ratio from the total series without stratification. As the age-specific estimates of risk ratio are identical, it is obvious that the ML procedure also gives $\hat{\rho}_r = 2.25$ and, therefore $\hat{\rho}^* = 2.62/2.25 = 1.16$. Consider-ing the existence of confounding within the two 10-year categories of age, the total

TABLE 3

Venous thrombosis in relation to oral contraceptives (O.C.) use among hospitalized women (ref. 4)

O.C.	Age category								
	20–29 years			30–39 years			Total		
	Thrombosis			Thrombosis			Thrombosis		
	+	−	Total	+	−	Total	+	−	Total
+	10	39	49	2	14	16	12	53	65
−	18	158	176	12	189	201	30	347	377
Total	28	197	225	14	203	217	42	400	442
$\hat{\rho}$	2.25			2.25			2.62		

confounding by age might correspond to $\hat{\rho}^* = 1.3$ with the corresponding $\hat{\rho}_s = 2.62/1.3 = 2.0$.

DISCUSSION

Confounding and residual components in risk *difference* ("attributable risk")—the risk in the exposed minus that in the non-exposed—in cohort studies have been dis-cussed quite thoroughly by Kitagawa (5).

The present paper presents simple risk *ratio* measures of confounding and of the residual association between exposure and disease, both for cohort and case-control stud-ies. The measure of confounding ($\hat{\rho}^*$) follows immediately from the definition of the con-founding effect, provided that the "null" situation is not approached in the usual manner (where the marginal frequencies are "fixed") but by "fixing" those frequencies which generally do not materially depend on the effect of exposure (i.e., on the number of cases among the exposed). Consideration of cohort studies suggests that the most natural RR measure of the residual associa-tion might be the $\widehat{SMR}$, i.e., the sample standardized RR ($\hat{\rho}_s$) with the exposed series as the standard. This has conceptual appeal and makes the estimate of crude RR ($\hat{\rho}_c$) to have a simple multiplicative parti-tioning: $\hat{\rho}_c = \hat{\rho}^*\hat{\rho}_s$. And quite interestingly, it turns out that this residual parameter (SMR or ρ_s) can be estimated in a simple manner from case-control studies as well. The procedure adds a "summary relative risk" with a clear-cut interpretation to the several measures previously discussed by Mantel and Haenszel (6).

REFERENCES

1. Cornfield J: A method of estimating comparative rates from clinical data. Applications to cancer of the lung, breast and cervix. J Natl Cancer Inst 11: 1269–1275, 1951
2. Gart JJ: Point and interval estimation of the common odds ratio in the combination of 2 × 2 tables with fixed marginals. Biometrika 57: 471–475, 1970
3. The Boston Collaborative Drug Surveillance Program: Excess of ampicillin rashes associated with allopurinol or hyperuricemia. N Eng J Med 286: 505–507, 1972
4. Miettinen OS: Comprehensive monitoring of hospitalized patients in the evaluation of side-effects of oral contraceptives. Presented to the International Symposium on Statistical Problems in Population Research, the East-West Population Institute, Honolulu, August 1971
5. Kitagawa EM: Components of a difference between two rates. J Am Stat Assn 50: 1168–1194, 1955
6. Mantel N, Haenszel W: Statistical aspects of the analysis of data from retrospective studies of disease. J Natl Cancer Inst 22: 719–748, 1959

II–7.

Jerome Cornfield: Joint Dependence of Risk of Coronary Heart Disease on Serum Cholesterol and Systolic Blood Pressure: a Discriminant Function Analysis. Federation Proceedings 1962; 2:58–61.

The following paper by Jerome Cornfield helped introduce to epidemiology the concept of using multivariate models to overcome the limits of "thinness of data" encountered in ordinary stratified analysis. The model employed (given in equation 5 of the article) is now commonly known as the multiple logistic model, and has become one of the primary tools of epidemiologic analysis.

The method used by Cornfield to derive the model and estimate its parameters was introduced in an earlier paper by Cornfield, Gordon, and Smith [1961], and is based on an assumption of multivariate normality of the risk factors within disease groups. This is an unrealistic assumption in general, and this method was soon rendered obsolete by the development of estimation methods based on less restrictive assumptions (e.g., Walker and Duncan [1967]). Nevertheless, it is instructive to work through Cornfield's derivation as an illustration of the connection between disease-specific risk factor distributions and multivariate risk functions.

More importantly, Cornfield's discussion of the *interpretation* of the fitted model's parameters is still valid, and his careful exercise in translating the parameter estimates into relative risk estimates remains a paradigm for proper use of modeling results. My only criticism here is that he did not mention the possibility that the very large relative risk estimated for the joint effect of cholesterol and blood pressure may have been an artifact of employing the logistic model, as the model can force relative risk estimates to be spuriously large when comparing risk at extremes of risk factor values or combinations. This problem can be circumvented by comparing risks within more typical values of the risk factors, and by checking results against those obtained from stratified analysis. Apparently, the problem and its solution were not well recognized before the 1970's, but are discussed by Gordon in the next article.

References:
Cornfield J, Gordon T, Smith WW. Quantal response curves for experimentally uncontrolled variables. Bull Int Statist Inst 1961; 38:97–115.
Walker SH, Duncan DB. Estimation of the probability of an event as a function of several independent variables. Biometrics 1967; 54:167–179.

Joint dependence of risk of coronary heart disease on serum cholesterol and systolic blood pressure: a discriminant function analysis

JEROME CORNFIELD

Biometrics Research Branch, National Heart Institute, Bethesda, Maryland

THE ASSOCIATION BETWEEN increased risk of coronary heart disease and elevated levels of serum cholesterol and systolic blood pressure is well known. Several questions about the magnitude of this association remain unanswered, however. Thus, are there critical values of serum cholesterol (or blood pressure) below which no relation between disease risk and cholesterol value exists, but which when exceeded are accompanied by abrupt elevations in risks? If no critical value exists is it nevertheless true that a given elevation is associated with a larger "effect" when added to a high rather than a low level? Does the apparent effect of serum cholesterol persist when levels of systolic blood pressure are held constant, and does the apparent blood pressure effect persist when serum cholesterol is held constant? If they do, are the effects independent of each other or do they, in the sense of the pharmacologist, potentiate each other?

Answers to these and related questions offer no difficulty in principle. They require continued observation of the frequency with which coronary heart disease develops in a well-defined population, for each member of which measurements of the magnitudes of possible risk factors have been made. Several such longitudinal studies are now in progress. The present analysis is based on the long-term follow-up study of heart disease in Framingham, Massachusetts (2). The results discussed were obtained from clinical examination of a sample of 1,329 of the male population (aged 40–59) of the town carried out from September 1948 through August 1952 and from their subsequent follow-up over a 6-year period. During this period 92 of the original sample developed clinically manifest coronary heart disease (myocardial infarction or angina pectoris). The combination of these two conditions into a single category is not, of course, intended to imply that they necessarily have the same etiology.

Table 1 shows the ratio of number of new events to number of men exposed for different combinations of serum cholesterol and systolic blood pressure after 6 years of follow-up. Certain qualitative conclusions emerge from an examination of this table. Thus, for those with serum cholesterols below 200 mg/100 cc the associated disease risk increases from 2 new cases in 6 years out of 119 exposed at systolic blood pressures below 127 mm Hg to 4 out of 26 at pressures above 167 mm Hg. A similar increase in risk with increasing blood pressure is suggested for the other levels of serum cholesterol shown. In the same way for those with blood pressures below 127 mm Hg the 6-year risk increases from 2/119 for those with cholesterol levels below 200 to 7/74 for those with cholesterol levels above 260. A similar increase in risk with increasing cholesterol level is suggested for each of the other blood pressure groups shown.

Simple inspection of the results is thus sufficient to suggest certain qualitative conclusions—the absence of a critical value for either cholesterol or blood pressure and the persistence of at least some association with each variable when the value of the other is held constant within broad limits. The thinness of the data nevertheless imposes a clear limit to the kinds of conclusions that this form of analysis will support. Inspection of the coarse groupings of Table 1 is, for example, hardly sufficient to indicate the way in which the effects of cholesterol level and blood pressure combine to influence the risk of the disease. Because of these limitations and because additional information will accumulate only slowly, one is led to seek a more searching form of analysis than simple inspection. The use of a mathematical model which summarizes the observations in a small number of disposable parameters seems to offer the only present hope of obtaining quantitative answers to questions of interest.

The model that we use is that of discriminant functions (1, 4), but because our objective is not that of discriminating between two populations, it is useful to start with a brief description of the method, emphasizing those aspects most important for the present application.

We begin with the case of one variable and consider as two separate populations those who did (CHD) and did not (NCHD) experience a new coronary event during the study period. Each of these populations is characterized by a frequency distribution with respect to the variable being considered. Thus, the CHD frequency distribution is such that the estimated proportion with serum cholesterols below 200 mg is 12/92, whereas NCHD frequency distribution is such that the estimated proportion with serum cholesterols below 200 mg is 307/1237. The essential characteristic of the method of discriminant functions is that for the observed frequencies one substitutes a mathematical formula describing a theoretical frequency distribution. The particular theoretical distribution used should, of course, be compatible with the observations and should be completely characterized by the values of a small number of disposable parameters, such as the mean or standard deviation.

Deferring the choice of distribution momentarily, suppose that the proportion of CHD individuals with serum cholesterols between Y and $Y + h$ can be adequately described by some simple function which we denote by $f_1(Y)h$, when h is reasonably small, while that for the NCHD population is $f_0(Y)h$. Denote the proportion of the combined populations who belong to the CHD population by p ($= 92/1329$). Finally, introduce the risk function, $P(Y)$, which denotes the proportion of individuals with serum cholesterol of Y who belong to the CHD population. Then elementary algebraic manipulation, or an application of Bayes' formula (3), is sufficient to show that

$$P(Y) = 1/[1 + (1 - p)f_0(Y)/pf_1(Y)] \qquad (1)$$

Thus, if theoretical frequency distributions can be found which adequately characterize the CHD and NCHD populations, then the risk function can be deduced from *equation 1*. An excellent description of both Framingham CHD and NCHD distributions with respect to cholesterol is provided by the log normal distribution. That is to say, in both populations log cholesterol has a normal distribution (Fig. 1 of ref. 1).

If f_0 and f_1 in *equation 1* are replaced by appropriate expressions for normal frequency distributions with different means but the same standard deviation, it is easy to show that

$$P = 1/[1 + e^{-(\alpha + \beta X)}] \qquad (2)$$

where

$X = \log_{10}$ cholesterol
$\beta = (\mu_1 - \mu_0)/\sigma^2$
$\mu_1 =$ mean $\log_{10}$ cholesterol for the CHD population
$\mu_0 =$ mean $\log_{10}$ cholesterol for the NCHD population
$\sigma^2 =$ the common variance of $\log_{10}$ cholesterol
$\alpha = -\log_e (1 - p)/p - \beta[(\mu_0 + \mu_1)/2]$

The curve (2) is S shaped, starting at $P = 0$ and increasing up to a level of $P = 1$. In the range of observations made up to now, e.g., with P less than one-fourth, the full sigmoid appearance is not apparent and the curve appears exponential. For many purposes it is convenient to express *equation 2* in the linear form:

$$\log_e P/(1 - P) = \alpha + \beta X \qquad (3)$$

The effect of inequality of the variances in the two populations, an inequality not suggested by present

TABLE I. *Ratio of Number of New Events in 6 Years to Number Exposed to Risk by Initial Systolic Blood Pressure and Serum Cholesterol*

Serum Cholesterol, mg/100 cc	Blood Pressure, mm Hg				
	Total	<127	127–146	147–166	167+
Total	92/1329	20/408	28/555	20/224	24/142
<200	12/319	2/119	3/124	3/50	4/26
200–219	8/254	3/88	2/100	0/43	3/23
220–259	31/470	8/127	11/220	6/74	6/49
260+	41/286	7/74	12/111	11/57	11/44

Framingham results, is to add a third term to the right-hand side of *equation 3* of the form γX^2, where

$$\gamma = \frac{1}{2}\left(\frac{1}{\sigma_0^2} - \frac{1}{\sigma_1^2}\right) \qquad (4)$$

(and to change the value of α).

The same analysis applies to the single variable, systolic blood pressure, except that the frequency distribution of log blood pressure is not quite normal. This can be seen by plotting on probability paper the cumulative frequencies against log blood pressure. The curve is not linear, as it would be if normality applied. The plot against the logarithm of (blood pressure -75) is linear, however, so that if Y denotes blood pressure, $\log_{10}(Y - 75)$ has a normal frequency distribution for both CHD and NCHD populations.

To consider both the cholesterol and systolic blood pressure variables simultaneously, it is sufficient to find frequency distributions in the two variables which characterize both CHD and NCHD populations. If a frequency distribution in a single variable is thought of as a curve in which frequency is plotted against X, then a bivariate frequency distribution can be thought of as a surface in which the frequency is plotted against the values of both variables, say X_1 and X_2. Empirical analysis of the Framingham results indicates that both CHD and NCHD populations are described by bivariate normal frequency functions in $\log_{10}$ cholesterol and $\log_{10}$ (blood pressure -75) with differing means but having equal variances and correlation coefficient (section 9 of ref. 1).

The equivalent of *equation 2* is then:

$$P = 1/[1 + e^{-(\alpha + \beta_1 X_1 + \beta_2 X_2)}] \qquad (5)$$

where

$X_1 = \log_{10}$ cholesterol
$X_2 = \log_{10}$ (blood pressure -75)

and α, β_1, and β_2 are easily computed functions of the means of log cholesterol and log (blood pressure -75) of the CHD and NCHD population, and of the variances of the two variables and correlation coefficient between them. The linear version of *equation 5* is

$$\log_e P/(1 - P) = \alpha + \beta_1 X_1 + \beta_2 X_2 \qquad (6)$$

Formulas for approximate confidence limits on the coefficients β_1 and β_2 are available (formula 7.8 of ref.

1). The right-hand side of *equation 6* is usually referred to as the discriminant function (α is often omitted), since its numerical value may discriminate between those likely and unlikely to become members of the CHD

TABLE 2. *New CHD in 6 Years Follow-Up: Actual and Expected Number of Cases Among Men 40–59*

Serum Cholesterol, mg/100 cc	Systolic Blood Pressure, mm Hg	New CHD		Population at Risk
		Expected*	Actual	
200	Total	10.5	12	319
	<117	0.8	2	53
	117–126	1.4		66
	127–136	1.8	2	59
	137–146	2.3	1	65
	147–156	1.6	2	37
	157–166	0.7	1	13
	167–186	1.4	3	21
	187+ over	0.5	1	5
200–209	Total	5.9	2	133
	<117	0.5		21
	117–126	0.8	2	27
	127–136	1.4		34
	137–146	1.0		19
	147–156	1.0		16
	157–166	0.7		10
	167–186	0.4		5
	187+ over	0.1		1
210–219	Total	6.9	6	121
	<117	0.4		15
	117–126	0.9	1	25
	127–136	1.0	2	21
	137–146	1.5		26
	147–156	0.4		6
	157–166	0.9		11
	167–186	1.1		11
	187+ over	0.8	3	6
220–244	Total	22.3	23	334
	<117	0.6		20
	117–126	2.9	8	69
	127–136	4.7	2	83
	137–146	5.5	6	81
	147–156	2.4	3	29
	157–166	1.5	1	15
	167–186	3.1	2	27
	187+ over	1.6	1	10
245–259	Total	11.6	8	136
	<117	0.5		14
	117–126	1.3		24
	127–136	2.3		33
	137–146	2.0	3	23
	147–156	1.9	2	19
	157–166	1.3		11
	167–186	0.7	2	5
	187+ over	1.5	1	7
260–284	Total	16.0	23	156
	<117	1.0	1	22
	117–126	1.4	5	22
	127–136	2.1	2	26
	137–146	3.5	2	34
	147–156	1.9	4	16
	157–166	1.7	2	13
	167–186	2.7	6	16
	187+ over	1.5	1	7

TABLE 2.—*Continued*

Serum Cholesterol, mg/100 cc	Systolic Blood Pressure, mm Hg	New CHD		Population at Risk
		Expected*	Actual	
285+ over	Total	18.9	18	130
	<117	0.7		11
	117–126	1.7	1	19
	127–136	3.1	4	28
	137–146	3.1	4	23
	147–156	2.8	1	16
	157–166	2.5		12
	167–186	3.2	3	14
	187+ over	1.9	1	7

* Expected number of cases = (population at risk)/[1 + $e^{(23.13 - 6.14 X_1 - 3.29 X_2)}$].

population. Our present interest is not in discrimination in this sense, but in using *equation 6* to study the quantitative nature of the dependence of risk on serum cholesterol and systolic blood pressure levels. If the variances and correlation coefficients of the CHD and NCHD populations had been unequal three terms would have been added to the right-hand side of *equation 6* of the form $\gamma_1 X_1^2 + \gamma_2 X_2^2 + \gamma_3 X_1 X_2$.

Granting the bivariate normal model, all the data on which Table 1 is based can then be summarized in the six constants α, β_1, β_2, γ_1, γ_2, and γ_3, and the answers to any questions about the joint dependence of risk on cholesterol and blood pressure levels are contained in them. Because of the near equality of the observed variances and correlation coefficient in the two populations the last three constants can be treated as zero. The estimates for the other three are: $\beta_1 = 6.14$ (3.35–9.00), $\beta_2 = 3.29$ (1.75–4.88), and $\alpha = 23.13$, where the numbers in parentheses are 95% confidence limits. Table 2 compares the actual and expected number of new CHD cases obtained on this basis. The agreement appears satisfactory.

The following approximation simplifies the subsequent discussion. When the value of P is small (say < 1/5), log $P/(1 - P)$ can be written as log P,* in which case it is easy to verify (remembering that logs of cholesterol and blood pressure are to base 10) that

$$P = .0091 \left(\frac{Y_1}{100}\right)^{2.66} \left(\frac{Y_2 - 75}{100}\right)^{1.47} \tag{7}$$

where Y_1 and Y_2 are serum cholesterol (in mg/100 cc) and systolic blood pressure (in mm Hg). The confidence limits on the exponents are from 1.45 to 3.90 and 0.76 to 2.12.

We may now return to the questions with which we started. It is clear first of all that the description provided by *equation 7* is incompatible with the idea of a critical value for either cholesterol or blood pressure. Although the notion of decision values, e.g., of 260 mg for cholesterol or 160 mm Hg for systolic blood pressure, may be

* For some of the values of X_1 and X_2 observed, P considered as the 6-year risk is too large for this approximation to be entirely accurate. For the 1-year risk, which is one-sixth of the 6-year risk, the approximation holds for all observed X_1 and X_2.

convenient clinically, these values are not associated with abrupt changes in risks.

Rather than ask about critical values, however, we may ask how the change in risk associated with changes in either variable depends on the level from which the change takes place. This includes the question of critical values as a special case. It is important here to distinguish between absolute and relative changes. Because both exponents in *equation 7* exceed unity, a given absolute increase in either variable will be associated with a larger absolute increase in risk when the change takes place from a high rather than a low level. A given difference in milligrams per 100 cc of cholesterol will thus be associated with a larger absolute difference in risk when added to a large rather than a small initial level. A similar conclusion applies to systolic blood pressure, except that since the lower 95% confidence limit is below unity, it is less certain.

The conclusion is different, however, if one considers percentage changes. Because of the form of *equation 7* a given percentage difference in cholesterol is associated with the same percentage difference in risk no matter what the level to which the difference is added. A 1% difference in cholesterol is associated with a 2.66% difference in risk throughout the range of cholesterol values. If one would lower cholesterol levels by a given amount, say 15%, and if *equation 7* describes not only the association between risk and cholesterol level in Framingham, but also the change in risk that would accompany an experimental alteration in serum cholesterol, then the relative risk would be $(.85)^{2.66}$, or a reduction of about 35%. This would be true no matter what the level of cholesterol from which the 15% reduction occurred.

Because of the subtractive 75 in systolic blood pressure, given percentage changes in blood pressure are associated with larger percentage changes in risk when starting from low than from high blood pressure. A 1% difference in systolic blood pressure will be associated with a percentage difference in risk of $1.47\ Y/(Y - 75)$, where Y is the starting level. Thus, at a starting blood pressure of 110 mm Hg a 1% difference in blood pressure is associated with a 4.62% difference in risk. This contrasts with a starting level of 175 mm Hg, where a 1% difference is associated with a 2.57% difference in risk.

For both cholesterol and blood pressure the form of *equation 7* implies that the percentage effect on risk of a given percentage change in either variables is independent of the level of the other variable. No matter what the blood pressure a 1% difference in cholesterol is associated with a 2.66% difference in risk. A 1% increase in systolic blood pressure from 110 mm Hg is associated with a 4.62% difference in risk no matter what the cholesterol level. Finally, from *equation 7* the effect of simultaneous differences in blood pressure and cholesterol on percentage differences in risk is multiplicative. A simultaneous 1% change in cholesterol and in blood pressure from a starting level of 110 mm Hg will result in a relative risk of $(1 - .0266)(1 - .0462)\%$. A useful way of summarizing these relations is by considering the percentage difference in risk associated with cholesterol values at the 5th and 95th percentiles, with blood pressures at the 5th and 95th percentiles, and with both cholesterol and blood pressure at their 5th as compared with their 95th percentiles. These are summarized below:

	Risk 95th Percentile Relative to 5th Percentile
Cholesterol alone (166–301 mg)	4.8
Blood pressure alone (110–177 mm)	4.8
Both	23.4

The population in the upper 5% of either the cholesterol or blood pressure distribution has a risk more than 4.8 times as large as that in the lower 5%, while individuals who are in the upper 5% with respect to both (about ¼ of 1% of the population) have a risk more than 23.4 times as large as those who are in the lower 5% with respect to both.

SUMMARY

1) Discriminant functions have been used to describe the relationships in the Framingham population between risk of developing coronary heart disease, serum cholesterol level, and systolic blood pressure.

2) Critical values of either variable, at which sharp increases in risk occur, were not found.

3) A 1% difference in serum cholesterol is associated with a 2.66% difference in risk at all levels of serum cholesterol.

4) A 1% difference in systolic blood pressure is associated with a 4.62% difference in risk at blood pressures of 110 mm Hg and of 2.57% at 175 mm Hg.

5) There is an almost fivefold difference in risk between the upper and lower 5% with respect to serum cholesterol or systolic blood pressure alone, and an almost 25-fold difference between those who are in the upper 5% of the population with respect to both variables and those who are in the lower 5% with respect to both.

REFERENCES

1. CORNFIELD, J., T. GORDON, AND W. W. SMITH. *Bull. Intern. Statistical Inst.* 38: 97, 1961.
2. KANNEL, W. B., T. R. DAWBER, A. KAGAN, N. REVOTSKIE, AND J. STOKES III. *Ann. Internal Med.* 55: 33, 1961.

3. PARZEN, E. *Modern Probability Theory and Its Applications.* New York: Wiley, 1960, p. 119.
4. RAO, C. R. *Advanced Statistical Methods in Biometric Research.* New York: Wiley, 1952.

II–8.

Tavia Gordon: Hazards in the Use of the Logistic Function.
Journal of Chronic Diseases 1974; 27:97–102.

While the introduction of multivariate models undoubtedly gave the epidemiologist a power-ful tool, every powerful tool has its hazards. Tavia Gordon was an appropriate person to warn of hazards in the use of the logistic model, as he had overseen much of the logistic analysis of the Framingham study. He begins here with a discussion about a now-settled issue, the choice between discriminant-function (Cornfield) and maximum-likelihood (Walker-Duncan) estimates of the logistic parameters. The rapid advances in computers since 1974 have rendered the discriminant-function estimates unnecessary and obsolete. They have also made it easier to heed Gordon's warnings about the strict assumptions inherent in the logistic model: it is now possible to fit and compare alternatives to the logistic model, via programs such as GLIM [Baker and Nelder, 1978]. Nevertheless, Gordon's advice that "cross-classification is the method of choice for explor-ing the inadequacies of the multiple logistic function" remains true, and applies to other models as well. I believe Gordon's succinct editorial should remain essential reading in epidemiologic statistics for a long time to come.

Reference:
Baker RJ, Nelder JA. General linear interactive modeling (GLIM), release 3. Oxford: Numerical Algorithms Group, 1978.

J Chron Dis 1974, Vol. 27, pp. 97–102. Pergamon Press. Printed in Great Britain

Editorial

HAZARDS IN THE USE OF THE LOGISTIC FUNCTION WITH SPECIAL REFERENCE TO DATA FROM PROSPECTIVE CARDIOVASCULAR STUDIES

(*Received* 9 *July* 1973)

SUPPOSE we are interested in examining the relation of CHD (coronary heart disease) incidence to the level of systolic blood pressure. The most direct approach is to measure blood pressure in a population of interest, group individuals of nearly similar systolic pressures, and observe the subsequent CHD incidence (within a specified period of time) in each of these groups. If we do this, we are likely to find that groups of persons with higher pressures tend to have higher incidence but that this is not a completely smooth trend. As the number of persons under observation increases, the trend can be expected to become smoother. Where it is not possible to sufficiently increase the number of observations to accomplish the desired amount of smoothing, it is sometimes appropriate to smooth the observations by some form of statistical graduation.

A common method of graduation with data from prospective cardiovascular studies is the logistic function. In the univariate case, each person in the sample of individuals under study is estimated to have a probability of the event expressed as $y(x)=[1+e^{-(a+bx)}]^{-1}$. In the instance cited, x is a specific systolic pressure at baseline and $y(x)$ is the probability that a person will develop CHD during a specified duration of follow-up given that he has the pressure. To graduate the data using this function, it is necessary to estimate only two parameters. Very frequently the smoothed results seem quite consistent with the unsmoothed rates obtained from categorical analysis.

There are two methods in use for estimating the logistic parameters. One, proposed by Cornfield [1], yields explicit solutions by a minor but ingenious modification of linear discriminant analysis [2]. The other, proposed by Walker and Duncan [3], is an iterative procedure involving less restrictive assumptions than the discriminant-based estimates. Since it is a least-squares estimate, by that criterion it provides better estimates. However, it is computationally more expensive and sometimes it will not converge to a solution.

Conceptually, the two estimating procedures involve different rationales. Discriminant analysis assumes that there are two different populations, one sick, the other well. As formulated by Cornfield, these two populations are assumed to be normal, with equal variances (or, in the multivariate case a common variance–

covariance matrix [4]) but different means. Even where these assumptions are obviously incorrect, the graduation usually fits the data fairly well. Sometimes, and especially when the independent variable is discontinuous, however, the fit is very unsatisfactory. What is worse, there appears to be no method to predict when a very bad fit will occur [5].

While any procedure leading to a bad fit is inherently suspect, it must be remembered that the analytical use of this function, particularly in the multivariate case, can logically be regarded as a form of discrimination and the robustness of this procedure is well-demonstrated. Moreover, it is our own experience that the discriminant-based estimates and Walker–Duncan ones may yeild similar tests of significance for the parametric estimates, even where the estimates themselves are quite different.

The maximum likelihood estimation, on the other hand, is based on the concept of a dose-response. The higher the blood pressure (dose), for instance, the greater the CHD incidence (response). The Walker–Duncan procedure yields satisfactory fits, even where the independent variable is discontinuous. Moreover, the total estimated incidence (the sum of $y(x)$ for all x in the sample) is constrained to the total actual incidence. In discriminant-based estimates this is not true, and the resultant estimates are occasionally very bizarre; for example, the estimated number of cases may be far in excess of the actual number of cases. In addition, discriminant-based procedures seem to have a slight tendency to overestimate the higher conditional probabilities. But these are exceptions: discriminant-based estimates generally provide quite satisfactory graduation.

If the logistic function were applied only to the univariate case, it would be of minor interest. So long as the incidence is fairly low (which is usually the case) reasonable graduation over the central range of the independent variable can be achieved by a variety of methods including unweighted linear regression. The chief value of the logistic function in the univariate case lies in providing an estimate of the gradient of incidence on the independent variable and an estimate of the standard error of that estimate. This leads to a test of significance based on the full use of the available detail.

It is the multivariate case where the logistic function has yielded a rich bonus in the analysis of cardiovascular data. The reasons for this are obvious. If continuous variables are partitioned along their scale and several such variables are cross-classified, the number of cells in the resultant table quickly multiply. For example, 5 continuous variables divided into thirds along their range yields a table with 243 cells. Not only is it rare to have enough incidence cases to occupy that many different cells, it is rare to have populations large enough for that purpose. Moreover, where there is a distinct gradient of risk along a variable, a very broad class will include individuals with quite distinct conditional probabilities of the event.

The practical and theoretical limitations to the use of cross-classification in evaluating relationships of this sort has made a multiple logistic model exceedingly attractive. This model is constructed in the same form as the univariate: $y(x)=[1+e-(a+\Sigma b_i X_i)]-1$, where i is the index for the n independent variables entered into the calculation. Instead of calculating the incidence rates for a large number of cells and attempting to see the picture, it becomes possible to graduate the data by estimating the limited number of parameters in the multiple logistic function. If the shape of the n–dimensional curve has been correctly judged to be logistic, we have achieved not only a good fit of the data, but are in a position to estimate the confidence we can place in this fit.

As in linear regression, a graduation to one set of data cannot be expected to fit another set of data as well. Thus, the ability to predict CHD from a multivariate logistic function (which in the jargon of cardiovascular epidemiology has come to be called a 'risk function') is not usually as good as the fit to the original data would suggest. At the same time, there is a countervailing consideration, namely, the biasing effect of error in the measurement of the independent variable. In the univariate case, using the discriminant-based estimates, technical variation independent of other sources of variation will inevitably lead to an understatement of the expected magnitude of the regression coefficient. The argument for this conclusion is identical with that for linear regression [6].

The synthetic uses of the logistic function, substituting a combination of observable variables (say, blood pressure and serum cholesterol levels) for an unobservable variable (say, the subsequent development of CHD), are fairly clearcut. When such uses are being considered, the statistical manipulations can be quite mechanical and still be useful. Arbitrary step-down or step-up methods may be used to select an efficient subset of variables for identifying 'high risk' individuals (that is, persons whose conditional probabilities are higher than average). Considerations of cost and convenience can be entered into the calculation either formally or informally. The multiple logistic function has proved very useful for cardiovascular screening and will probably be used increasingly for that purpose [7].

However, it is probably its analytical value that has most attracted investigators. Statistical analysis, in the context of the present discussion, can be defined as a process of disentangling the contributions of a set of variables to some outcome. It is imbued with semantic confusion between subject-matter logic and statistical logic. Even its primary statistical aspects have numerous hazards.

The model assumptions themselves are a source of hazard. The logistic model we have used assumes a linear combination of the independent variables. This assumption is not always warranted. For example, the logistic regression of CHD on serum cholesterol or cigarette smoking decreases with age and is different for men and women. In statistical terms, there are interactions among these four independent variables. To enter the independent variables as linear terms into a multiple logistic function, ignoring this interaction, misrepresents the data. The safest way to explore questions of this sort is to revert to cross-classification.

Interaction is, of course, one of the central concerns of statistical analysis. Consider a specific example. Two of the most important precursors to congestive heart failure (CHF) are CHD and hypertension. We might, conceivably, construct a multiple logistic function with CHD (a dichotomous variable) and age and systolic blood pressure (continuous variables) as the independent variables and the probability of CHF as the dependent variable. Suppose, however, that the onset of CHD alters the relation of both blood pressure and age to CHF. The multivariate logistic function proposed may produce a very powerful synthetic 'predictor' but lead to completely misleading analytical conclusions.

The alternative, in this case, is very simple; namely to estimate separate logistic functions for persons with and without CHD. This partly categorical analysis is feasible because nearly half of the CHF incidence is preceded by CHD. Where data are too skimpy for such a categorical approach, we must forbear drawing analytical conclusions based on the apparent general adequacy of the fit. Ironically, then, while the multiple logistic function is used to repair the inadequacies of analysis by cross-classification, cross-classification is the method of choice for exploring the inadequacies of the multiple logistic function.

Where the interaction can be represented by some simple algebraic device (say, a cross-product term), it may be helpful to enter such a term into the exponent. Of course, when the decision to use a term is based on a prior evaluation of the sample data, it becomes difficult to evaluate the test of significance for this term, but this is really of less concern than the appropriateness of the graduation. However, interactions may be too complex, particularly when the number of variables is fairly large, to be described adequately by a single multiple logistic function. It might also be noted that discriminant-based estimation is not designed to represent non-linear terms. Efforts to use it for that purpose are apt to lead to nonsensical results in cases where the results of Walker–Duncan estimations are quite reasonable.

Another difficult fitting problem arises where the conditional probability is not monotonic in the independent variable. If, for example, incidence is high both for low body weights and high body weights, and low for intermediate weights, the logistic function may not provide a good fit to the data. In general, adding a quadratic term to the exponent is to be avoided and alternative methods of exploring such relationships should be sought.

In brief, the multiple logistic operates satisfactorily if the assumption of a linear exponent is more or less correct. Under these conditions, a modest amount of data can be graduated with considerable assurance. In such a case, however (as in other multivariate analysis), it is practically impossible to test the appropriateness of the assumptions. In effect, we must rely on other evidence (or our hopes) for assurance that the procedures used are relevant. By the same token, where there are relatively few observations of either the independent variable or the dependent, at very high or very low blood pressures, for example, the assumption that the graduation holds has no means of confirmation within the sample data.

Frequently, the analytical interest focuses on a single variable and the concern is to make due allowance for other associated variables in evaluating the one variable of interest. Suppose we are interested in the relation of diabetes to the incidence of congestive heart failure. We know that diabetes is correlated with blood pressure, which in its turn is strongly associated with the incidence of congestive heart failure. Hence, the use of the multivariate technique to control the nuisance variable (in this instance, blood pressure) in order to assess the net effect of diabetes. Whether it is sensible to approach the analysis this way must be based on subject matter considerations. To the extent that blood pressure is controlled by glucose tolerance, the question may not be definable at all.

To take another case in point. Suppose serum cholesterol, blood pressure and relative weight are entered as independent variables in a multiple logistic function with CHD as the dependent variable. It is most likely that the coefficient for relative weight, which may be statistically significant by itself, will approach zero in this multivariate context. What does that mean? It certainly does not *per se* mean that relative weight is unimportant. It may rather mean that its effect is intermediated by blood pressure and serum cholesterol levels. In any case, the question is a subject-matter one, not a statistical one.

A similar difficulty arises when two highly correlated variables are included; for example, both systolic and diastolic pressures. When this is done, the calculations become very unstable and may, in fact, be uninterpretable. If the multivariate function is used synthetically, this is no problem. If the interest is analytic, it is ordinarily best to delete one of these twins before proceeding or to repeat the analysis first with one, and then the other. Similar problems sometimes arise when interaction terms, which are bound to be highly correlated with the parent linear terms, are added to the function.

What is more, the relation of a variable to some outcome depends on the other independent variables included in the set of characteristics under consideration. It is not at all uncommon to have a coefficient which is significant in the univariate case become indistinguishable from zero in the multivariate case. The same thing may happen when we shift from one multivariate set of variables to another. Nor is the effect of adding a variable to the set always to reduce the coefficients assigned to the original variables. Thus, there is never a unique multivariate conclusion. The only general guide is that where a conclusion respecting association of a variable in the multivariate case is not consistent with what is found in the univariate case, great care must be exercised in drawing conclusions.

The specificity of multivariate analysis makes any process of looking for an optimum subset of variables very chancy. If a synthetic function is being sought, this is not a serious problem. If the function is being used analytically to discern which variables are important, this is a most serious reservation.

Persons familiar with multiple linear regression will recognize in slightly altered form many of the same cautions and concerns. That being the case one final caution might be worth making and that is that analogies between the two should not be pushed to an extreme. For example, since the dependent variable is dichotomous, the testing of goodness of fit is not entirely straightforward and can only be approximated by breaking the estimated function along its range and comparing the actual number of cases in each class with the sum of the estimated probabilities. The analog to variance analysis which has been proposed to answer the same question is very tenuous at best.

It must be said, finally, that no method of analysis can redress a shortage of information from prospective studies. It is, of course, this very shortage which provides the most powerful motive for using (and sometimes misusing) the multivariate logistic function. It is the shortage of information that impels analysts, for example, to combine data for all age groups and both sexes into one grand analysis, often without even a preliminary exploration of the problems this may entail. The power and elegance of the logistic function make it an attractive and flexible statistical instrument, but in the end, we cannot push a button and hope that everything will come out all right. Because frequently, it will not.

TAVIA GORDON

Biometrics Research Branch,
National Heart and Lung Institute,
National Institutes of Health,
Bethesda, Maryland, U.S.A.

REFERENCES

1. Cornfield J, Gordon T, Smith WW: Quantal response curves for experimentally uncontrolled variables. **Bull Int Sta Inst XXXVIII:** Part III, 97–115, 1961

TAVIA GORDON

2. Fisher RA: The use of multiple measurements in taxonomic problems. **Ann Eug Lond** 7: 179–188, 1936
3. Walker SH, Duncan DB: Estimation of the probability of an event as a function of several independent variables. **Biometrics** 54: 167–179, 1967
4. Truett J, Cornfield J, Kannel W: A multivariate analysis of the risk of coronary heart disease in Framingham. **J Chron Dis** 20: 511–524, 1967
5. Halperin M, Blackwelder W, Verter J: Estimation of the multivariate risk function: a comparison of the discriminant function and maximum likelihood approaches. **J Chron Dis** 24: 125–158, 1971
6. McNemar Q: **Psychological Statistics.** New York, Wiley, 1949, pp. 134–136
7. Gordon T, Kannel WB: Multiple contributors to coronary risk: Implications for screening and prevention. **J Chron Dis** 25: 561–565, 1972

II–9.

Paul R. Sheehe: Dynamic Risk Analysis in Retrospective Matched Pair Studies of Disease.
Biometrics 1962; 18:323–341.

I am indebted to James Schlesselman for bringing to my attention Paul Sheehe's 1962 paper "Dynamic Risk Analysis of Retrospective Matched Pair Studies of Disease." I believe the paper contains several innovations that were ignored because they were too far ahead of their time. It is therefore presented, out of sequence, along with articles of a comparable level of evolution.

On page 327 of this paper, Sheehe proposed to analyze case-control studies by means of "risk functions" (actually hazard functions in modern failure-time analysis terminology—what Sheehe termed "risk" would now be known as "incidence density" or "hazard"). On pages 330–331 he introduced a relative risk model, based on multiplicative interactions and exponential dose-response for the factors, that is analogous to the modern Cox and conditional logistic models. On page 332, he illustrated the univariate version of this model as a special case of a general relative risk function. On the same page, he delineated what is now known as matched density sampling as a foundation for the application of his model. On pages 332–334, he showed that the effect parameter in his model can be estimated from matched density-sampled case-control data, and can be taken as a coefficient in a linear model for the log relative risk. Finally, on pages 338–339, he considered the possibility of other dose-response models, especially linear models.

The paper is not without problems, especially on page 326, where Sheehe erroneously omitted the step of dividing by length of time interval when deriving his "instantaneous incidence" or "risk" measure. Note that in failing to do so, Sheehe's interval incidence necessarily converges to zero as the interval width converges to zero. Fortunately, this error does not affect the rest of the paper, for Sheehe mathematically treated his "risk function" as if it were a properly derived hazard function. Also, Sheehe's least-squares statistics would now be regarded as obsolete in light of modern conditional-likelihood methods. But all in all I suspect our current methods would be far more advanced had Sheehe's work been properly recognized in its time.

(Nonstatistical readers be warned: Sheehe's paper is the most technically difficult of this collection.)

Reprinted from
BIOMETRICS
THE BIOMETRIC SOCIETY, Vol. 18, No. 3, September 1962

DYNAMIC RISK ANALYSIS IN RETROSPECTIVE MATCHED PAIR STUDIES OF DISEASE

PAUL R. SHEEHE

Roswell Park Memorial Institute,
Buffalo, New York, U. S. A.

SUMMARY

It has been shown how a general population model of an exponentially changing risk of disease may be tested against retrospective matched pair data. In the illustrative analysis of breast cancer data it was found that the risk of breast cancer increased exponentially at a greater rate during menstrual years than during other phases of life.

Analysis of proportional risk functions and linear risk functions, as well as the extension of exponential risk functions to more than one variable, were discussed.

INTRODUCTION

Retrospective studies of disease are so called because the investigator observes an effect, that being a number of individuals with and without the disease, and "looks back" into the histories of the diseased cases and non-diseased controls for an explanation of the effect. If the relative frequency of some characteristic is sufficiently greater among the cases than among the controls, then the characteristic may be an indicator of disease.

The principal reason for looking backward at the problem is evident when the alternative prospective approach is considered. In a prospective, or forward looking, study a chosen number of individuals with the characteristic is compared with a chosen number without the characteristic to see if the relative frequency of disease in the two classes is different. But if disease is infrequent, as is generally true, either very large samples or a very long follow-up period, or both, would be required in order to obtain reliable frequencies of disease. The retrospective study short circuits this problem, but in accomplishing this it presents problems of its own. There is of course the very practical problem of obtaining histories of individuals—memories are faulty and records may be missing or inaccurate. But assuming the historical data to be adequate, there is the added problem of interpretation.

TABLE 1
POPULATION DISTRIBUTION

	With Characteristic	Without Characteristic	Total
With disease	N	N'	$N + N'$
Without disease	M	M'	$M + M'$
Total	$N + M$	$N' + M'$	$N + N' + M + M'$

While one may "look back" by practical necessity, one prefers to "think forward" for theoretical purposes. It is preferable to ask whether the risk of disease is greater for individuals with the characteristic, to reason from causes or antecedent conditions to effects, rather than the reverse.

Cornfield [1951] showed that the retrospective study is amenable to a prospective interpretation when he considered a situation similar to that schematized in Table 1. Table 1 shows a population consisting of four classes of individuals. There are N individuals who have both a certain characteristic and the disease, M with the characteristic but not the disease. Among those without the characteristic there are N' and M' respectively with and without disease. Among those with the characteristic, the relative frequency, or prevalence, of disease is

$$P_1 = N/(N + M).$$

This is assumed to be very low. Similarly, for those without the characteristic, the prevalence is

$$P_2 = N'/(N' + M'),$$

also assumed to be very low. Thus, the prevalence of disease among those with the characteristic, relative to those without, is

$$R = \frac{N}{N + M} \bigg/ \frac{N'}{N' + M'} = \frac{N(N' + M')}{N'(N + M)}$$

There is a second expression which closely approximates the relative prevalence. This expression is the relative odds. Among those with the characteristic the odds for disease are N/M. Among those without, the odds are N'/M'. The relative odds are therefore

$$(N/M)/(N'/M') = NM'/N'M.$$

Since the disease is rare, N and N' are relatively small, so that

$$(N' + M')/(N + M) \simeq M'/M.$$

Hence, the expression for relative prevalence reduces approximately to the relative odds,

$$R \simeq \frac{NM'}{N'M}.$$

Under the retrospective method of study, a relatively large fraction, f, of diseased cases are sampled, and a much smaller fraction, g, of non-diseased controls are sampled. Ignoring any sampling error for the moment, the number of sampled cases with and without the characteristic is

$$n = fN \quad \text{and} \quad n' = fN',$$

and

$$m = gM \quad \text{and} \quad m' = gM',$$

respectively. Then the relative odds computed from the retrospective data are

$$\frac{nm'}{n'm} = \frac{NM'}{N'M} \simeq R.$$

That is to say, the retrospective method has not disturbed the relative odds, and the relative odds, in turn, closely approximate the relative prevalence in the population.

Relative incidence can be dealt with in a retrospective study in similar fashion by defining the population differently. Instead of a population of individuals with and without disease, a population wholly free of the disease is initially defined. As before, this population is divided into those individuals with and without a certain characteristic. In either of these two classes of the population, incidence is defined as the proportion of individuals who come down with the disease within a specified interval of time. The situation is again represented by Table 1, except that now the population is considered to be initially free of the disease, and now the class "With disease" should be taken to mean "With disease at some time during the specified interval", also, "Without disease", should be taken to mean "Without disease throughout the specified interval". The subsequent manipulations of cell frequencies apply equally well to this situation. Ignoring sampling error, as before, and assuming that the incidence of disease is low, the relative odds this time approximate relative incidence instead of relative prevalence.

The problems of sampling error and the combination of relative odds have been dealt with recently by Woolf [1954] and by Haldane

[1955]. In addition, an interesting method of estimation in retrospective studies of matched cases and controls has been demonstrated by Kraus [1960]. While these methods all pertain to dichotomous characteristics, this paper will deal with certain risk functions of *measured* variables which can be tested in retrospective matched pair studies. The method to be developed will be illustrated with data from a study of breast cancer cases and matched controls.

1. RISK FUNCTIONS OF AGE

As shown in the introduction, either a relative prevalence or a relative incidence interpretation can be obtained from retrospective data when populations appropriate to each interpretation are defined and sampled. This paper will deal more directly with relative incidence than with relative prevalence. However, it will deal with incidence in a multiplicity of classes, rather than just two classes. These classes will be defined according to age, among other variables.

In order to obtain some notion of the nature of these age-specific classes, consider some large population of females. Each of the individuals will live free of breast cancer, for example, for a certain number of years. Therefore, we can visualize classes of all the individuals alive and free of past or current history of breast cancer at age 0, 1 year, 2 years, and so on. (Note that these classes are not mutually exclusive with respect to individuals. The same individual may appear in many classes.) The one-year incidence of breast cancer among 0 year olds is, by definition, the number of individuals coming down with breast cancer in the one year interval following birth, divided by the number of 0 year olds. Similarly, the 1 year incidence is defined for every age class. An individual who survives one year without breast cancer enters (as in a life-table) a new age class at the end of the year. Thus, we can visualize the passage of an individual from one age class to the next throughout her lifetime until either breast cancer or death occurs. But age classes need not be limited to annual increments. Half year incidences could be considered for classes specified at every half year of age. Indeed, the age interval, and correspondingly the interval over which incidence is observed, may be made very small. For theoretical purposes, we postulate, finally, an instantaneous incidence, which we call risk, for every instant of age. Thus, at any defined age instant in the breast cancer-free lifetime of an individual, that individual belongs to a class with a certain postulated risk (instantaneous incidence) of breast cancer. This postulated risk is introduced here as a convenience in overcoming the difficulty of expressing a large number of hypothesized short-interval incidences.

As will be done later in the study of breast cancer, it may be postulated that risk is some integrable function of age. This postulated risk function, when weighted by the number of individuals at each instant of age can be summated over a specified interval to yield an hypothesized number of new cases of breast cancer in that interval*. When this number is divided by the size of the class at the beginning of the age interval, an hypothesized incidence is obtained. Thus, there is a direct connection between risk functions and hypothesized age-specific incidence in the population. This connection establishes the meaning of risk functions of age. In the following section, a risk function will be constructed as a model of the development of breast cancer in the lifetimes of individuals in the general female population. Subsequently, it will be shown how such a risk function can be brought to bear on retrospective data. Since risk functions of age have an immediate prospective connotation in terms of age-specific incidences in the population, the establishment of a connection between risk functions and retrospective data will provide a prospective interpretation of certain patterns of change observed in retrospective studies of disease.

2. CONSTRUCTION OF AN HYPOTHETICAL RISK FUNCTION FOR BREAST CANCER

Now, with some misgivings, we shall propose a model for the risk of breast cancer as it develops in the general female population. This model is something more than a shot in the dark because it does not seem to conflict in any obvious way with previous epidemiological findings. Yet we are almost certain that this model will sooner or later be found to err in one or many respects. Why, then, attempt any model at all? There are, we think, some good reasons. First by setting up an explicit mathematical model, its shortcomings become quite obvious to readers familiar with the complexity of the problem. This, we hope, minimizes any tendency for this study to be taken as "final" in any sense. But, second, setting up a model which is something more sophisticated than an ill-considered null hypothesis helps to provide a structure for subsequent study. And third, it is a fact that this model furnished the stimulus to develop an analytical procedure which may well have applications in the epidemiological study of many

---

*Let r_t be an integrable risk function of age, t. To find the hypothesized number of cases in a given time interval, denote the small component intervals between successive occurrences of death or breast cancer by $k = 0, 1, .., D$, such that $\sum_{k=0}^{D} \Delta t_k$ equals the duration of the defined interval. Let l_k be the class size during each component interval. Then

$$S = \sum_{k=0}^{D} l_k (\int r_t dt)_k$$

is the hypothesized number of new cases occurring during the interval.

other diseases.   We therefore ask the reader to make allowances for our naivete in attempting a bald mathematical model in the face of so complex a problem.

With what is known now of the epidemiology of breast cancer, many hypotheses might be formed, but the most promising line seems to be some hypothesis connecting breast cancer with ovarian function. Lilienfeld [1955, 1956] found that the age-specific incidence of breast cancer rose exponentially with age for both single and married women up to approximately age 40 or 45, corresponding roughly with age at menopause.   From that age on, the incidence continued to rise, but at a definitely lower rate of increase.   Moreover, the break in the rise was somewhat postponed for single women.   Further study uncovered the fact that the average age at menopause for single women was later than for married women.   This was not because of later natural menopause for single women but rather because artificial menopause was much more frequent among married women.

In a combined review and international study of the epidemiology of breast cancer, Wynder et al., [1960] discussed these and other consistent factors which have been observed in studies of the disease, such as: the more frequent occurrence of breast cancer among single than among married women; the later age of marriage of breast cancer patients; the reduced incidence of breast cancer brought about by pregnancy, or events subsequent to pregnancy, such as nursing; the reduced frequency of breast cancer among castrated women; and an increased incidence presumably due to prolonged ovarian activity, i.e. late menopause.   In addition to these factors related to marriage and hormonal functioning, cognizance was taken of "background" variables such as heredity, familiality, race, religion, and socio-economic status, each of which may play its own etiological role.   But the basic conception which the authors developed was that "any factor that can reduce endocrine function (through its effect on menstruation) tends to reduce the risk of developing breast cancer".

In relation to endocrine function, five phases of a woman's life can be identified: (1) pre-menarchal; (2) menstrual; (3) pregnancy; (4) lactation; (5) post-menopausal.   In general, the conception expressed by the authors reviewed above could be interpreted to mean that a long menstrual history would be indicative of high risk of breast cancer, while long histories of the other four phases lead to a relatively lower risk of breast cancer.   In view of Lilienfeld's results, it would seem plausible to relate the risk of breast cancer to an exponential function of years spent in each phase of life.   Thus, it might be hypothesized that risk of breast cancer increases exponentially as menstrual years increase, while the increase is not so rapid or the risk even diminishes exponentially during the other phases. The rate of increase or decline in risk might be different for each of the five phases, and indeed, if we were to specify phases in more detail, the risk function might be exceedingly complex. But in the interest of simplicity and feasibility of testing the hypothesis, it seems desirable to confine our hypothesis within the limits of these five phases.

The preceding paragraph contains the most general form of the breast cancer model which we shall adopt. That model is, simply, that the risk of breast cancer at any moment, under certain conditions which will be specified, is an exponential function of the number of pre-menarchal, menstrual, pregnancy, lactation, and post-menopausal years lived by a woman up to that moment. When we refer to a "woman's risk" at a given moment, we mean that at a given moment the woman belongs to the general class of all women free of breast cancer after a certain number of years spent in each type of phase, and we refer to the risk for that class. If the woman is in the menstruating phase, then "her risk", so to speak, changes with each passage of time to that of the class of women with a longer history of menstruation. If the woman is in another phase, then "her risk" changes with each passage of time to that of the class of women with a longer history in that phase.

According to the model, risk may be increasing or decreasing at a constant exponential rate during any given phase of life. The rate of change may be different in each of the five phases of life. But both for practical and expository purposes, we now make a simplifying assumption. We shall assume that the rate of change is the same in pre-menarchal, lactating and post-menopausal phases. This is not to say that we prefer this over letting the pre-menarchal and lactating years "ride free". There seems to be some evidence in the literature that lactation furnishes some added retardation of the risk of breast cancer, and little is known about how risk may change during the pre-menarchal years. But in the United States at least, there is little variation in the age of menarche, this being usually somewhere between 12 and 14 years, and there is even less variation in lactating years, since relatively few women have nursed more than 10 months during their lives. Therefore, the error, if any, of assuming the same rate of change in risk during these phases as during the post-menopausal phase will be of about the same relative magnitude for most women. Subsequently, when we come to compare the hypothesized risk of a breast cancer patient (i.e., the risk of breast cancer in the class of women to which the breast cancer patient belonged just prior to diagnosis) with an age-matched control, the two errors will cancel out in the ratio of the two risks, if age of menarche and history of lactation are the same. If the menarche and lactation histories differ, they will usually differ only slightly, as indicated above, and unless the rates of change in risk during these two phases are radically different from that in post-menopausal years, the *relative* risk of case versus control will be affected only slightly. The simplifying assumption reduces the number of identified phases of life to three: (1) menstrual, (2) pregnancy, (3) other. For post-menopausal women, the principal source of variation in non-menstrual and non-pregnant years is, of course, the number of post-menopausal years.

In addition to phase of life, the growth or decay of risk may depend on certain "background" conditions for a defined class of women. Among the "background" conditions are such factors as age, race, country of birth, religion and marital status. No specific hypothesis is made here as to how risk of breast cancer may be affected by these background variables. It is considered that risk of breast cancer may or may not be affected by these factors. It is only hypothesized that risk of breast cancer is an exponential function of phase history for classes of women within specified age, racial, country of birth, religious and marital status groups.

In the illustrative analysis which will be presented, all the background variables mentioned above will be employed. In addition, to simplify the analysis, years of pregnancy will also be relegated to the background, so that we shall be directly concerned only with testing the exponential risk hypothesis with respect to variations in menstruating years and "other" years (excluding years of pregnancy). The exponential risk hypothesis is expressed precisely as follows:

$$r_{ix'x''} = C_i a_1^{x'} a_2^{x''}, \qquad i = 1, 2, \cdots, s,$$

where

   x' denotes number of menstrual years,

   x'' denotes number of other years (excluding pregnancy),

   a_1 and a_2 are constants relating the number of menstrual and "other" years, respectively, to risk,

   i denotes a class of women with a specified age, race, country of birth, religion, marital status, and pregnancy history,

   C_i is an unknown ith class constant,

and

   $r_{ix'x''}$ is the risk of breast cancer in the ith class of women in the sub-class denoted by variables x' and x''.

Thus, the hypothesized risk for the sub-class of women denoted by $(ix_1'x_1'')$, relative to the risk for another sub-class, $(ix_2'x_2'')$, is given by

$$R_{i12} = r_{ix_1'x_1''}/r_{ix_2'x_2''} = a_1^{x_1'-x_2'}a_2^{x_1''-x_2''}.$$

One final simplification results from the fact that in any relative risk comparison of two sub-classes in the ith class of women, age and years of pregnancy are constant. Hence the sum of menstrual and 'other' (excluding pregnancy years) is constant:

$$x_1' + x_1'' = x_2' + x_2'',$$

so that

$$(x_1' - x_2') = -(x_1'' - x_2'').$$

Consequently, the expression of the relative risk for two sub-classes reduces to

$$R_{i12} = a_1^{x_1'-x_2'}\cdot a_2^{-(x_1'-x_2')} = (a_1/a_2)^{x_1'-x_2'}$$
$$= b^{x_1'-x_2'}.$$

Since the relative risk for the two sub-classes of i has been reduced to an expression involving only menstrual years, we shall drop the prime notation. Through the remainder of this paper, the quantity x means menstrual years. Thus,

$$R_{i12} = b^{x_1-x_2},$$

is the hypothetical relative risk for two sub-classes of i, where b is some constant to be determined. The latter expression can be restated in the following form,

$$R_{i12} = e^{(x_1-x_2)\ln b},$$

or in a form which will be used later on,

$$\ln R_{i12} = (x_1 - x_2) \ln b.$$

Referring back to Lilienfeld's studies, if $\ln b$ were positive, this would be in general agreement with the greater slope in the plot of log incidence versus age during the generally pre-menopausal years than during the generally post-menopausal years.

Under the exponential hypothesis, or for that matter any other risk hypothesis expressed as a function of x, we are obviously dealing with a measured· variable. Moreover, the chosen risk function is a dynamic hypothesis in the sense that hypothesized risk changes with age. The problem which lies before us is to see how such an exponential risk function can be brought to bear on retrospective matched pair data. This problem is taken up in the next section, following which an illustrative analysis of the breast cancer hypothesis will be presented.

4. THE CONNECTION BETWEEN RISK FUNCTIONS AND RETROSPECTIVE MATCHED CASE-CONTROL PAIRS

Consider all non-diseased individuals at all points of time in the ith class. Within this class it is hypothesized that risk of disease is some function of x,

$$r_{ix} = f_i(x).$$

Thus, in the sub-class designated by ix_1 ,

$$r_{ix_1} = f_i(x_1),$$

and in ix_2 ,

$$r_{ix_2} = f_i(x_2).$$

Consequently, the relative risk for sub-class ix_1 versus ix_2 is

$$R_{i12} = f_i(x_1)/f_i(x_2),$$

For example, under the exponential hypothesis for breast cancer,

$$R_{i12} = b^{x_1-x_2}.$$

Now consider in detail the process of obtaining cases and matched controls. Let the number of individuals in the ix sub-class be denoted H_{ix} and the number of individuals in the ith class by K_i .

Also, let

$$H_{ix} = K_i L_{ix} ,$$

where L_{ix} is the relative distribution of x for individuals in the ith class.

Now, *as part of the hypothesis,* assume that the *conditional probability* that the next case which comes from class i will be from the ix sub-class is proportional to the number of individuals times the risk of disease in that sub-class:

$$P_{ix} = cH_{ix}r_{ix} ,$$

where c is some proportionality constant. Assume also that the matching control for the next case is obtained at random from the same class (i) as the case. Thus, the conditional probability (given i) of a control from an ix sub-class is

$$P_{x:i} = L_{ix} .$$

Then the probability of an x_1 case and x_2 control given that they are both in the ith class is

$$P_{i12} = cH_{ix_1}r_{ix_1}L_{ix_2} .$$

Similarly, the probability of an x_2 case and x_1 control (inverse pair) is given by,

$$P_{i21} = cH_{ix_2}r_{ix_2}L_{ix_1} .$$

The relative probability (odds) of an x_1x_2 pair versus the inverse pair x_2x_1 in the ith class is therefore

$$P_{i12}/P_{i21} = cH_{ix_1}r_{ix_1}L_{ix_2}/cH_{ix_2}r_{ix_2}L_{ix_1}$$
$$= cK_iL_{ix_1}L_{ix_2}r_{ix_1}/cK_iL_{ix_2}L_{ix_1}r_{ix_2}$$
$$= r_{ix_1}/r_{ix_2}$$
$$= R_{i12} .$$

That is to say, the relative probability (odds) of a given pair (ix_1 , ix_2) versus its inverse is equal to the relative risk for individuals in (ix_1) versus individuals in (ix_2). Finally, given that one individual in a matched pair is x_1 and the other is x_2 , and that they both come from class i, the conditional probability of an x_1 case and x_2 control is given by

$$R_{i12}/(R_{i12} + 1),$$

while the complementary probability of the inverted pair is given by

$$1/(R_{i12} + 1)$$

or, what is equivalent, by

$$R_{i21}/(R_{i21} + 1).$$

This connection between an hypothesized risk function of x and the retrospective matched pair method of collecting data is the key to the analysis of matched pair studies presented in the next section.

5. ANALYSIS OF THE EXPONENTIAL RISK HYPOTHESIS

Suppose that h matched pairs, $j = 1, 2, \cdots , h$, have been obtained in the manner already described. Denote by x_{j1} the higher measurement of x in the jth pair and by x_{j2} the lower measurement of x. The odds for the case having the higher measurement are given by R_{j12} , and the odds for an inverse pair (case lower than control) are given by R_{j21} , as discussed in the previous section. That is, the conditional probability of an x_1 case and x_2 control (obverse pair) is $R_{j12}/(R_{j12} + 1)$, while the conditional probability of an inverse pair is the complement, $1/(R_{j12} + 1)$. For example under the exponential risk hypothesis in the study of breast cancer, the relative risk of breast cancer in subclasses jx_1 versus jx_2 is

$$R_{j12} = b^{x_1 - x_2}.$$

Thus the odds for an obverse pair are

$$R_{j12} = b^{x_{j1} - x_{j2}}, \quad \text{where} \quad x_{j1} > x_{j2}.$$

Now the h pairs can be listed in rank order of the hypothesized odds for an obverse pair, or what is equivalent, in rank order of the *absolute* difference between x_{j1} and x_{j2}. Categories containing 15 or more neighboring pairs can be formed and the frequencies of obverse and inverse pairs in these categories can be counted.

Now we may obtain an estimate of the natural log relative risk in each of the categories. Haldane has shown [1955] that for a binomially distributed variable the natural logarithm of the ratio of P to Q can be estimated with negligible bias from a sample of a fixed size by adding $\frac{1}{2}$ to the observed frequencies and obtaining the natural log of the ratio of the two numbers. We may apply Haldane's results to the particular situation by noting that the category size is fixed, and that the number of obverse or inverse pairs is binomially distributed as a consequence of the model we have described. Thus, letting n_k equal the observed number of obverse pairs in the kth category and m_k equal the observed number of inverse pairs,

$$y_k = \ln [(n_k + \tfrac{1}{2})/(m_k + \tfrac{1}{2})]$$

is an approximately unbiased estimate of the natural log relative risk in the kth category. The variance of this statistic, worked out to a close approximation by Haldane in the same article, is given by

$$s_{y_k}^2 = \frac{1}{n_k + 1} + \frac{1}{m_k + 1}.$$

The above expressions will be used in our illustrative analysis of breast cancer cases and controls. (See columns 5, 6 and 7, Table 1.)

But by hypothesis, we also have the relative risk, R_{j12}, which equals the odds for an obverse pair, for every j. The hypothesized natural log relative risk is, therefore,

$$\ln R_{j12} = (x_{j1} - x_{j2}) \ln b = d_j \ln b.$$

(Note that d_j must be positive since $x_{j1} > x_{j2}$ by definition.) Within a given category, k, the average of hypothesized log relative risks is thus

$$(\overline{\ln R})_k = \bar{d}_k \ln b.$$

This average is slightly lower than the logarithm of the expected relative risk. This is because variation exists among the hypothesized log relative risks within the kth category. However, because the category contains neighboring hypothetical values, this variation is generally slight, and in any event the variation of hypothetical log relative risks within categories is minute in comparison to the random variation of observations. Thus, by hypothesis, we have that $\bar{d}_k \ln b$ is approximately equal to the natural log relative risk in the conditional domain defined by the observed values of x in k.

The model for the general population has been reduced to a linear model applicable to retrospective data. Consequently, we are in a position to analyze the variance of the observed log relative risks, obtain a least squares estimate of $\ln b$, test $\ln b$ for significance, and use the residual variation of observed log relative risk in a "goodness of fit" test of the model. This is illustrated in the next section.

6. ILLUSTRATIVE ANALYSIS

The data for this study come from hospital admissions to Roswell Park Memorial Institute from April 17, 1955 to April 17, 1957. The cases consist of all female breast cancer patients admitted during that interval. From the remaining females admitted without breast cancer or cancer of the genitals, a matching control for each case was selected at random from the class of admissions corresponding to the case with respect to age (5 year age groups), race (white, non-white), nativity (native, foreign-born), religion (Protestant, Catholic, Jewish), marital status (married, single) and parity (number of live births). The reader will note that there is only an approximate conformity between practical matching and theoretical concepts, particularly in connection with age and parity matching. Also the reader will appreciate the fact that a new opportunity for the risk hypothesis to go wrong has been introduced by the choice of hospital patients rather than a complete or random sample of the population. (Ideally, we mean the whole human population.) Let it suffice here to say that these are the practical problems which make the results of any single study inconclusive and which warrant attention in further studies. (See discussion.)

Table 2 shows the data for 331 case-control pairs divided into 22 categories, each (except the last) of size 15. A few pairs for which the difference between case and control patients was zero have been dropped. This was done because it is logically true that the relative risk in identical sub-classes must be 1, and therefore no data are required to establish this truth.

Column (2) shows the categorical limits of the *absolute* difference

TABLE 2

PAIRED BREAST CANCER DATA ACCORDING TO RANKED CATEGORIES OF ABSOLUTE CASE-CONTROL DIFFERENCES IN MENSTRUAL YEARS

(1) Category (k)	(2) Categorical Limits of Absolute Case-Control Differences (d_i) (menstrual years)	(3) Average Absolute Case-Control Differences ($\bar{d}_k$)	(4) Number of Pairs		(5) Observed Relative Risk $(n_k + \frac{1}{2})/(m_k + \frac{1}{2})$	(6) Observed Natural Log Relative Risk (y_k)	(7) Variance of y_k $\left[s_k^2 = \dfrac{1}{n_k + 1} + \dfrac{1}{m_k + 1} \right]$
			Obverse (Case > Control) (n_k)	Inverse (Case < Control) (m_k)			
1	0.1 to 0.7	0.36	9	6	1.46	.378	.243
2	0.7 to 1.0	0.91	8	7	1.13	.122	.236
3	1.0 to 1.1	1.01	7	8	0.88	-.128	.236
4	1.1 to 1.7	1.35	7	8	0.88	-.128	.236
5	1.7 to 2.0	1.83	6	9	0.68	-.386	.243
6	2.0 to 2.3	2.09	8	7	1.13	.122	.236
7	2.3 to 2.9	2.59	7	8	0.88	-.128	.236
8	2.9 to 3.0	2.99	4	11	0.39	-.942	.283
9	3.0 to 3.7	3.33	7	8	0.88	-.128	.236
10	3.7 to 4.1	3.97	7	8	0.88	-.128	.236
11	4.1 to 4.7	4.42	8	7	1.13	.122	.236
12	4.7 to 5.2	4.96	9	6	1.46	.378	.243
13	5.2 to 5.8	5.55	13	2	5.40	1.686	.404
14	5.8 to 6.3	6.04	9	6	1.46	.378	.243
15	6.3 to 7.0	6.85	11	4	2.56	.940	.283
16	7.0 to 7.9	7.59	12	3	3.57	1.273	.326
17	7.9 to 9.0	8.55	9	6	1.46	.378	.243
18	9.0 to 10.7	9.82	9	6	1.46	.378	.243
19	10.7 to 12.0	11.40	9	6	1.46	.378	.243
20	12.0 to 14.0	13.08	12	3	3.57	1.273	.326
21	14.0 to 16.3	15.05	11	4	2.56	.940	.283
22	16.3 to 27.7	21.99	12	4	2.78	1.023	.276
	TOTAL		194	137			

between case and control. Note that the range of variation is usually less than 1 year within a given class, the only exceptions being at the high end of the scale.

The average *absolute* difference, $\bar{d}_k$, between cases and controls has been entered in the third column. It is important to note that the average absolute difference is used, because it has been shown that the hypothesized natural logarithm of relative risk in these categories is proportional to $\bar{d}_k$, not the average of signed differences. The factor of proportionality is ln b which is to be estimated from the data.

In column (4) we have the observed number of obverse and inverse pairs, and from this is calculated the entries in columns (5), (6) and (7). Note that there is a general tendency for the observed relative risk and natural log relative risk in columns (5) and (6), respectively, to increase as $\bar{d}_k$ increases. The analysis of computed chi-squares is shown in Table 3.

The component of variation due to the least-squares estimated slope is highly significant and the residual is far from significantly large. This means that the exponential hypothesis has passed the test. Variations from hypothesis in the "goodness of fit" test of the model are of the very same magnitude as would be expected of random variations, as shown by the residual chi-square of 17.061 with 21 degrees of freedom. Also, more detailed inspection of deviations in the various categories reveals no meaningful pattern. At the same time the value of ln b has been found to be significantly different from 0, with a probability less than .0001.

The least squares estimate of ln b is given by

$$\sum w_k y_k \, \bar{d}_k / \sum w_k \, \bar{d}_k^2 = +.058.$$

It is positive, as hypothesized. The standard error of ln b is given by

$$1/\sqrt{\sum w_k \, \bar{d}_k^2} = .014.$$

TABLE 3

Analysis of Variance of Log Relative Risk*

Component of Variation	S. S.	d. f.	Probability
Total ($\sum w_k y_k^2$)	34.829	22	
Due to Slope [$(\sum w_k y_k \bar{d}_k)^2/\sum w_k \bar{d}_k^2$]	17.768	1	$<.0001$
Residual	17.061	21	$>.50$

*$w_k = 1/s_k^2$

Thus, approximate 95% confidence limits put the differential rate of change in risk of breast cancer during menstruating phases, as compared to "other" phases, somewhere between +3.1% and +8.5% per year. This is analogous to a person paying somewhere between an extra 3.1% to 8.5% in continuously compounded interest on a loan, except that here the accumulation is in terms of the risk of breast cancer.

7. DISCUSSION

Several questions arise in connection with the foregoing analysis. Among these are questions dealing with risk functions of other than exponential form, extensions to more than one variable, and hospital selection. These will be discussed in this section.

It is evident that the exponential risk hypothesis was particularly convenient in the analysis of retrospective matched pair data on breast cancer. The reader will recall that, once the risk function, r_{ix}, was specified, the door was opened to analysis by virtue of the fact that hypothesized relative risk in sub-class x_1 versus x_2 was given by

$$R_{i12} = r_{ix_1}/r_{ix_2} .$$

When r_{ix} is in the exponential form,

$$r_{ix} = C_i b^x,$$

the relative risk becomes

$$R_{i12} = b^{x_1 - x_2},$$

and

$$\ln R_{i12} = (x_1 - x_2) \ln b.$$

Since the natural logarithm of hypothesized relative risk is proportional to the difference between case and control measures of x, analysis of the natural logarithm of observed relative risk is quite simple.

While it is true that the exponential hypothesis for breast cancer seems to be appropriate in view of prior results such as Lilienfeld's, we can imagine other studies where it might make more sense to deal with, say, a linear risk function. The simplest non-null linear risk hypothesis might be one of proportionality:

$$r_{ix} = C_i x.$$

Then,

$$R_{i12} = x_1/x_2 .$$

Consequently, the conditional probability of an obverse pair would be given by

$$P_{i12} = \frac{x_1/x_2}{(x_1/x_2) + 1} = \frac{x_1}{x_1 + x_2}$$

and

$$Q_{i12} = 1 - P_{i12} = \frac{x_2}{x_1 + x_2},$$

is the probability of an inverse pair. In other words, x appears in the hypothetical probability expressions just as if it were an observed frequency rather than a measured variable. In this case, one could order all the observed pairs according to R_{i12} as the ordering principle, divide the array into a number of categories, count the number of obverse and inverse pairs in each category and test these observed frequencies against the hypothesized (expected) frequencies of obverse and inverse pairs in an approximate chi-square goodness of fit test. (When this is done with the breast cancer data, using x equal to menstrual years, the fit is rather poor, with P somewhere in the neighborhood of .10 to .03, depending somewhat on what rule is used to form the categories.) Chi-square here would have as many degrees of freedom as there are categories.

But under a more general linear hypothesis,

$$r_{ix} = C_i(a + bx),$$

the hypothesized relative risk is

$$R_{i12} = (a + bx_1)/(a + bx_2),$$

which evidently depends on the relative magnitudes of a and b. So, too, the conditional probabilities of obverse and inverse pairs would depend on the relative magnitude of a and b. In principle, it would be possible to specify the range of a/b such that the data fit the hypothesis within specified probability limits. But as a practical matter, such an analysis, which might require repeated chi-square tests, would be quite tedious unless an electronic computer were available. On the other hand, if the investigator were willing to develop a more specific hypothesis, in which the relative levels of a and b would be specified, then the analysis would reduce to the same type as under the proportionality hypothesis. This restriction in the applicability of the analysis seems to hold generally: in order to test risk hypotheses conveniently it appears desirable to reduce the hypotheses, possibly through specifying certain parameters, to either a proportionality or exponential function.

Note that we have dealt with testing non-null hypotheses. We can, of course, consider the null hypothesis as a particular case. Under the null hypothesis, however, the ordering principle on which categories are based is lost. No categories can be specified on this principle. But note that if we merely count the total number of obverse and inverse pairs and test the null hypothesis with one degree of freedom, we have a conventional sign test.

The exponential hypothesis seems to be most suited to the analysis because one not only obtains a goodness of fit test of the model, but at the same time obtains a test of the significance of the growth or decay constant. It is natural to wonder, therefore, whether the exponential hypothesis can be extended to more than one variable. That is, can hypotheses such as

$$r_{izv} = C_i a_1^x a_2^y$$

be tested?

Under this hypothesis, no difficulty is encountered in forming the relative risk:

$$R_{i12} = a_1^{x_1 - x_2} a_2^{y_1 - y_2}.$$

The natural logarithm of R_{i12} is a linear form

$$\ln R_{i12} = (x_1 - x_2) \ln a_1 + (y_1 - y_2) \ln a_2.$$

And so, if a suitable ordering principle can be specified so as to produce an array of pairs which can be classified into ordered categories, the analysis can proceed without difficulty. But this seems to be the big problem here, that no clear-cut ordering principle seems to be available. Unless the relative magnitude of a_1 and a_2 are somehow implied, one does not know in which order to place the pairs. Of course, it is sometimes possible to circumvent this difficulty in practical situations where one of the variables, say x, has an established relevance and the other does not. In this case, a null hypothesis with respect to a_2 can be entertained and the ordering principle becomes based on x alone. Then $\ln a_1$ can be estimated by the method illustrated in this paper. Then the pairs can be re-ordered according to $(y_1 - y_2)$ and classified into categories. Using the estimated value of $\ln a_1$, $\ln R_{i12}$ can be calculated for each pair and summed over all pairs in each category. Then a goodness of fit test of this null hypothesis can be made to see whether deviations of the number of obverse and inverse pairs are significantly great. Perhaps the most relevant component of chi-square in this test would be the linear component with respect to y. Also, perhaps, in some practical situations, this component of variation might be used to estimate $\ln a_2$. But such a method of estimation would clearly be subject to possible bias in the estimation of both a_1 and a_2.

The final question to be discussed is hospital selection. Customarily,

RISK ANALYSIS IN RETROSPECTIVE STUDIES **341**

if an hypothesis holds in the more general population of a city or state, it is taken to carry more weight than if it holds only in a hospital population. Of course, there is nothing sacred about a city or state-wide population, for there may well be selection in this population when reference is made to an even more general super-population extending further through time and space. But, as implied before, the burden of proof tends to pass to the counter-hypothesis (selection) when the original hypothesis holds repeatedly in a variety of circumstances. By the same token, results which have passed only a single test in a restricted situation such as a hospital should be viewed with some reserve.

The practical problem which arises is whether a hospital study provides a *prima facie* case for further studies on perhaps a larger scale. It seems that the case in favor of further study should generally be stronger when an hypothesis has passed a test even in a restricted setting. If, furthermore, the restricted study has shown agreement with a predicted *pattern*, as a result of a constructed risk function, then the case in favor of the hypothesis should be further strengthened. At least, since successfully predicted patterns of effects must tend to elicit comparably complex patterns from counter-hypotheses, an anonymous cry of "selection" will not suffice to explain away the results.

ACKNOWLEDGEMENTS

I wish to thank Dr. Morton L. Levin and Dr. Saxon Graham for their stimulating discussions and criticisms on both theoretical and practical levels, and to thank Mr. Oliver Glidewell for his assistance in the preparation of the data.

REFERENCES

Cornfield, J. [1951]. A method of estimating comparative rates from clinical data. Applications to cancer of the lung, breast and cervix. *Journal of the National Cancer Institute 2*, 1269–75.

Haldane, J. B. S. [1955]. The estimation and significance of the logarithm of a ratio of frequencies. *Annals of Human Genetics 20*, 309–11.

Kraus, A. S. [1960]. Comparison of a group with a disease and a control group from the same families, in the search for possible etiologic factors. *American Journal of Public Health 50*, 303–11.

Lilienfeld, A. M. and Johnson, E. A. [1955]. The age distribution in female breast and genital cancers. *Cancer 8*, 875–82.

Lilienfeld, A. M. [1956]. The relationship of cancer of the female breast to artificial menopause and marital status. *Cancer 9*, 927–34.

Woolf, B. [1954]. On estimating the relation between blood group and disease. *Annals of Human Genetics 19*, 251–3.

Wynder, E. L., Bross, I. J., and Hirayama, T. [1960]. A study of the epidemiology of cancer of the breast. *Cancer 13*, 559–601.

II–10.

Olli Miettinen: Estimability and Estimation in Case-Referent Studies. American Journal of Epidemiology 1976; 103:226–235.

Miettinen's "Estimability and Estimation in Case-Referent Studies" was the first (and for many years the only) published attempt to present a complete and coherent quantitative theory of estimation in case-control studies. The paper covers a lot of ground, and the reader is warned that it is probably the most dense and difficult of Miettinen's works. But this paper also marks the first appearance in mainstream epidemiologic literature of a good number of central concepts of modern case-control theory.

Perhaps most importantly, Miettinen carefully distinguished cumulative incidence (incidence as a proportion of a cohort falling ill, or "risk") from incidence density (cases per unit of person-time), a distinction that was known to pre-20th century epidemiologists but had become submerged in more recent times [Vandenbroucke, 1985]. Miettinen also delineated the types of case-control sampling schemes and assumptions needed to estimate ratios of the different types of incidence. In particular, he explicated the notion of incidence-density sampling (longitudinal sampling of controls over the case-incidence period) and showed that under certain conditions the odds ratio from density-sampled studies would estimate the incidence-density ratio, without the need of the rare disease assumption. Earlier work of Thomas [1972] and Kupper et al. [1975] had shown that under certain conditions cumulative incidence ratios could be estimated from odds ratios without the rare disease assumption; with the appearance of Miettinen's paper another link between the case-control odds ratio and rare diseases could be discarded.

But Miettinen's paper covers much besides odds ratios – he dealt with estimation of absolute rates, etiologic (attributable) fractions, and rate differences as well. The paper also includes one of Miettinen's more controversial innovations, the test-based principle of interval estimation. This principle was shown to be fallacious by Halperin [1977]. Although test-based intervals worked well enough with crude and Mantel-Haenszel odds ratios to become incorporated into case-control methodology in the years following their introduction, they can work quite poorly with other measures [Greenland, 1984]. Fortunately, ensuing statistical developments have rendered test-based limits unnecessary (e.g., see Kelsey et al., [1986], Rothman [1986]. For more recent results on the relation of prevalence to incidence, see Alho [1992] and Keiding [1991].

References:
Alho JM. On prevalence, incidence, and duration in stable populations. Biometrics 1992; 48:587–592.
Greenland S. A counterexample to the test-based principle of setting confidence limits. Am J Epidemiol 1984; 120:4–7.
Halperin M. Re: estimability and estimation in case-referent studies. Am J Epidemiol 1977; 105:496–498.
Keiding N. Age-specific incidence and prevalence: a statistical perspective. J Roy Stat Soc A 1991; 154:371–412.
Kelsey JL, Thompson WD, Evans AS. *Methods in Observational Epidemiology*. New York: Oxford, 1986.
Kupper LL, McMichael AJ, Spirtas R. A hybrid epidemiologic study design useful in estimating relative risk. J Am Statist Assoc 1975; 70:524–528.
Rothman KJ. *Modern Epidemiology*. Boston: Little, Brown, 1986.
Thomas DB. The relationship of oral contraceptives to cervical carcinogenesis. Obstet Gynecol 1972; 40:508–518.
Vandenbroucke JD. On the rediscovery of a distinction. Am J Epidemiol 1985; 121:627–628.

AMERICAN JOURNAL OF EPIDEMIOLOGY
Copyright © 1976 by The Johns Hopkins University School of Hygiene and Public Health

Vol. 103, No. 2
Printed in U.S.A.

ESTIMABILITY AND ESTIMATION IN CASE-REFERENT STUDIES

OLLI MIETTINEN

Miettinen, O. S. (Harvard School of Public Health, Boston, MA 02115). Estimability and estimation in case-referent studies. *Am J Epidemiol* 103: 226–235, 1976.

The concepts that case-referent studies provide for the estimation of "relative risk" only if the illness is "rare," and that the rates and risks themselves are inestimable, are overly superficial and restrictive. The ratio of incidence densities (forces of morbidity)—and thereby the instantaneous risk-ratio—is estimable without any rarity-assumption. Long-term risk-ratio can be computed through the coupling of case-referent data on exposure rates for various age-categories with estimates, possibly from the study itself, of the corresponding age-specific incidence-densities for the exposed and nonexposed combined —but again, no rarity-assumption is involved. Such data also provide for the assessment of exposure-specific absolute incidence-rates and risks. Point estimation of the various parameters can be based on simple relationships among them, and in interval estimation it is sufficient simply to couple the point estimate with the value of the chi square statistic used in significance testing.

biometry; statistics

The principles that currently govern epidemiologic thinking as to the fundamentals of case-referent (case-"control") studies do not apply to the most common type of such study in chronic-disease epidemiology. Here the principles are extended to encompass this kind of study. A simple, general-purpose statistical approach is also proposed. The results presented are generally self-evident, but some explanations are offered in appendix 1.

1. The classical principles

1.1. Essence. The prevailing principles concerning the estimability of parameters in case-referent studies derive from a classical paper by Cornfield (1). The principles might be expressed as follows (1, 2): First, the ratio of the odds of developing the

Received for publication April 3, 1975, and in final form July 23, 1975.

From the Departments of Epidemiology and Biostatistics, Harvard School of Public Health, and Department of Cardiology, Children's Hospital Medical Center, Boston, MA 02115.

Supported by Grants 5 P01 CA 06373 and HE 10436 from the National Institutes of Health.

illness for the exposed as compared to the non-exposed equals the ratio of the odds of having been exposed, contrasting cases of the illness to a reference series, and therefore the illness-odds ratio contrasting the exposed to the non-exposed is estimable from case-referent studies; and second, this parameter is approximately equal to the risk ratio when the illness is rare. The rationale is as follows (1, 2): Given risks of illness $R_1 = A/(A + C)$ and $R_0 = B/(B + D)$ for exposed and non-exposed people, respectively, the odds ratio for the illness is $[R_1/(1 - R_1)]/[R_0/(1 - R_0)] = AD/BC = (A/B)/(C/D)$. The last formulation for the odds ratio for illness between the exposed and the non-exposed reveals the identity of this parameter with the odds ratio for past exposure between cases and non-cases. Obviously, the ratio A/B is estimable from a series of cases, and C/D can be estimated from a reference (comparison, "control") series. Finally, the odds ratio parameter can be seen to equal the risk ratio (R_1/R_0) itself on the condition that $(1 - R_0)/(1 - R_1) = 1$, and this condition obtains with good approximation if the illness is rare.

1.2. Applicability. Upon careful appreciation of that rationale it is apparent that the classical principles of estimability apply, as such, to a particular type of case-referent study only. This special type is the one in which the subjects are ascertained at or after the *end of the entire risk-period* of interest. Such studies, though commonplace in acute-disease epidemiology, are rare in the chronic-disease field. (A conspicuous example is, however, the study of teratogenesis by means of ascertaining malformed and healthy newborns and comparing their exposure-histories in reference to the period of organogenesis.)

If formulated in terms of prevalence rather than risk, the classical rationale for estimability in case-referent studies also implies that studies based on *prevalent* cases provide for the estimation of *prevalence*-odds ratio; and when the prevalences are low, this parameter is practically interchangeable with the *prevalence* ratio itself.

The classical rationale does not, however, bear on the ordinary type of case-referent study in chronic-disease epidemiology—the type of study in which ascertainment occurs before the individual risk-periods are over, and in which incident rather than prevalent cases are enrolled.

2. The nature of the study

For a given exposure and illness, the objectives of a case-referent study are basically no different from those of a follow-up ("cohort") study. Thus, with reference to populations it is desired to learn about *rates* of occurrence of the illness in relation to the exposure (possibly in causal terms), within categories of age and other characteristics; and for individuals the concern is with *risks* (for various time periods) of the development of the illness in relation to the exposure, conditional on age and other characteristics.

The defining features of case-referent studies are that a series of people with and another without the illness are enrolled, and that their profiles with respect to the exposure, past or present, are ascertained and compared.

The internal validity of the study involves the following components: a) validity of selection: the probability of ascertainment is uninfluenced by the exposure history or status itself; b) validity of observation: lack of misclassification between cases and non-cases (referents, comparands, "controls") and between exposed and nonexposed; and c) validity of comparison: the use of a reference entity (usually diagnostic category) unrelated to the exposure, and the control of confounding.

3. Incidence density

3.1. The parameters. Incidence density ("force of morbidity" or "force of mortality")—perhaps the most fundamental measure of the occurrence of illness—is the number of new cases divided by the population-time (person-years of observation) in which they occur. For scientific purposes this measure is more meaningful if the experience of only actual candidates for the illness are considered in defining the population-time, i.e., if prevalent cases are not counted as contributing to the follow-up experience. For example, the incidence density of death is more meaningfully—and routinely—expressed in reference to follow-up experience with the living rather than with the living and the dead combined. In these terms, then, for the exposed described in figure 1 the incidence density (ID_1) in the time interval from t' to t'' is defined as

$$ID_1 = a''/C(t'' - t') \qquad (1)$$

instead of $ID_1 = a''/(A + C) (t'' - t')$. For the nonexposed, similarly,

$$ID_0 = b''/D(t'' - t'). \qquad (2)$$

It follows that the incidence density ratio (IDR) relating the exposed to the nonexposed is

$$IDR = (a''/b'')/(C/D), \qquad (3)$$

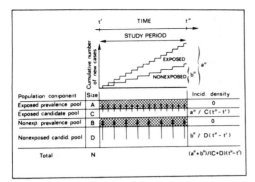

FIGURE 1. Static population (e.g. a particular age-group) over the time-span of a case-referent study based on *incident* cases. The sizes of the different component populations remain static, but there is turnover of membership in each compartment. The arrows indicate occurrences of new cases, i.e., transitions from the candidate pools to the prevalence pools. Note that the incidence-densities are zero in each of the prevalence pools, and that the incident cases are referred to the follow-up experiences in the candidate pools only. Also note that the incidence-density ratio is $(a''/b'')/(C/D)$, with a''/b'' and C/D estimable from the (incident) cases and referents, respectively, regardless of the levels of incidence or prevalence.

while the other relative measure, incidence density difference (IDD), is

$$IDD = (a''/C - b''/D)/(t'' - t'). \quad (4)$$

3.2. Estimability of ratio. In a case-referent study involving incident rather than prevalent cases, the cases (a exposed and b non-exposed) provide for the estimation of a''/b'' (as a/b), and C/D is estimable from the reference series (as c/d, the ratio of the sample numbers of exposed and non-exposed referents from the total pool of candidates for the illness). Consequently, the incidence density ratio is estimable from such studies; and in particular, no rarity-assumption is required for this. If the study is based on prevalent rather than incident cases, then it is necessary to assume that the duration of the illness is unrelated to the exposure.

3.3. Estimability of absolute parameters and difference. If the overall incidence density, for the exposed and the non-exposed combined, is known, then case-referent data provide for the estimation of the exposure-specific values and, thereby, for the estimation of the difference measure of relative occurrence (IDD). Even though this is well known, the prevailing principles of this estimation (1, 2) require added specificity as well as extension.

Sometimes a case-referent study involves complete ascertainment of new cases (over a particular time period) in a well-defined population of known size ($N = A + B + C + D$; cf. figure 1) (3, 4). If the reference series (of size n) is drawn from the total source populations, i.e., *without excluding prevalent cases* in the ascertainment, then it is always feasible to estimate C (as cN/n) and D (as dN/n) and therefore ID_1 and ID_0 themselves (cf. formulas 1 and 2) as well as their difference. No rarity-assumption is involved in this. In (the usual) instances in which the reference series is (unnecessarily) confined to non-cases, this type of estimation of ID_1 and ID_0 is feasible if it is realistic to assume low prevalence ($(C + D)/N \doteq 1$).

When those conditions do not obtain, it still is commonplace to have *a priori* knowledge about the overall incidence density (ID) for the exposed and non-exposed combined (for various categories of age and sex). Ordinarily, however, the overall incidence density is not known in the proper terms, with prevalent cases excluded in the computation of the population-time of experience. When this is the case, the reference series should again be drawn without excluding prevalent cases, and the proper incidence density (ID) may then be estimated from the available, improper value (ID^*) as

$$\hat{ID} = (ID^*)n/(c + d), \quad (5)$$

where n is the size of the reference series from the age category at issue, and $c + d$ is the size of the unaffected subgroup of it.

Given an estimate of the overall incidence density, whether from the study itself or from an outside source, the separate estimates for the exposed and nonexposed can usually be determined from the relations

$$ID_1 = (IDR)\,(ID)\,(1 - EF) \qquad (6)$$

and

$$ID_0 = (ID)\,(1 - EF), \qquad (7)$$

respectively, where EF is the etiologic fraction (proportion of all cases) related (or perhaps even attributable) to the exposure. The IDR is estimable as already discussed, and the EF has (5) the structure of

$$EF = [(IDR - 1)/(IDR)]\,(ER_1), \qquad (8)$$

where ER_1 is the exposure rate among incident cases (i.e., $ER_1 = a''/(a'' + b'')$). This approach is applicable when the association between the exposure and the illness is non-negative in the data ($\widehat{IDR} \geq 1$). Otherwise one may use the relationships

$$ID_1 = (IDR)\,(ID)/(1 - PF) \qquad (9)$$

and

$$ID_0 = (ID)/(1 - PF), \qquad (10)$$

where PF is the preventive fraction related to the exposure. It may be estimated (5) through the expression

$$PF = (1 - IDR)\,(ER_1)/[(1 - ER_1)\,(IDR) + ER_1]. \qquad (11)$$

4. Cumulative incidence-rate and risk

4.1. The parameters. Even though the source population of subjects tends to constitute a (dynamically) static group in each category of age (figure 1), with new people continually entering it at the lower bound (and within the range) of age and others exiting it (within the range and) at the upper bound, the data from successive age categories may be used to make inferences about an aging cohort of fixed membership and homogeneous, though continually increasing, age.

With regard to such an age-cohort, the interest is, firstly in the cumulative incidence of the group as it passes from one age to another, and, secondly, in the corresponding risks of its individual members. The cumulative incidence-rate for a span

of age is the proportion of the group developing the illness in that period, while the risk for an individual is the probability of his developing the illness in the particular span of age.

As a function of incidence density (ID) of first episodes of the illness (among those who never had it), the cumulative incidence-rate (CIR) for the age span a' to a'' is (6), given survival from other illnesses,

$$CIR_{a',a''} = 1 - \exp\left[- \int_{a'}^{a''} (ID_a)\,da\right]. \quad (12)$$

If age is discretized, then the cumulative incidence-rate (conditional on survival) over successive categories j' through j'' has the approximate expression of

$$CIR_{j',j''} \doteq 1 - \exp\left[-\sum_{j=j'}^{j''}(ID_j)w_j\right], \quad (13)$$

where w_j is the width of the jth category. When the cumulative incidence-rate is small, say less than 10 per cent, it may be reasonably approximated as

$$CIR_{a',a''} \doteq \int_{a'}^{a''} (ID_a)\,da \qquad (14)$$

or as

$$CIR_{j',j''} \doteq \sum_{j=j'}^{j''}(ID_j)w_j. \qquad (15)$$

Risk (R, for an individual) is the expected value of the cumulative incidence-rate (for a group):

$$R_{a',a''} = E(\widehat{CIR}_{a',a''}) \qquad (16)$$

4.2. Estimability of ratio. The estamability of cumulative incidence and risk from case-referent data is dependent, through the above relationships, on the estimability of incidence density.

The ratio of instantaneous risks is identical to the ratio of the corresponding incidence densities (cf. formula 15), so that the *instantaneous* risk ratio is estimable (through the exposure-odds ratio of incident cases) without any rarity-assumption in reference to either incidence density or prevalence.

For a *longer span of age*, from the beginning of category j' to the end of category j'', the risk ratio (assuming survival from other illnesses) is somewhat complicated: Even if the risk over that age span for both the exposed and the non-exposed is low enough to justify the use of formula 15, the corresponding risk ratio (RR) approximation is

$$RR_{j',j''} \doteq \sum_{j=j'}^{j''} (ID_{1j})w_j / \sum_{j=j'}^{j''} (ID_{0j})\,w_j$$

$$\doteq \sum_{j=j'}^{j''} W_j\,(IDR_j) / \sum_{j=j'}^{j''} W_{j'} , \qquad (17)$$

where $W_j = (ID_{0j})w_j$, and where the subscripts 1 and 0 refer to the exposed and the non-exposed, respectively, as before. Thus, the (point) estimation of the risk ratio over several categories of age, even when the risks themselves over that age span are small, involves the computation of a weighted average of the age-specific density ratios; and what is more, the weights involve the actual incidence densities of the non-exposed or at least numbers proportional to these. The determination of the weights can pose a serious problem, although the relationships in equations 7 and 10 tend to be very helpful. If the risks are not "low," then it is necessary to compute the ratio directly from the exposure-specific estimates of absolute risk.

4.3. Estimability of absolute parameters and difference. The exposure-specific risks over several age-categories, together with the corresponding risk differences, are in principle estimable through the application of formula 13. This requires that the overall age-specific incidence densities, for the exposed and non-exposed combined, are estimable from the data or known *a priori*, so that exposure-specific incidence densities are estimable within the categories of age (see section 3).

5. Prevalence rate

As was already noted, a case-referent study based on prevalent cases provides for the estimation of prevalence-odds ratio; and if the prevalence rate is low among both the exposed and the non-exposed, then the prevalence-odds ratio is approximately equal to the prevalence ratio itself.

This principle allows the estimation of (age-specific) ratio measures of relative prevalence with great ease, both conceptual and procedural.

But when a case-referent study is based on incident cases, as it usually is, inference about the relative prevalence among the exposed and the non-exposed involves some subtlety. Consider first a closed population with a static profile over time as to age-distribution etc. People make transitions from the candidate pool to the prevalence pool, and from the prevalence pool either back to the candidate pool or out of the population through death (figure 1). The static state is characterized by an equilibrium between the inceptions of new cases and the terminations of prevalent ones. Specifically, in a population of size N, the equilibrium prevalence rate PR, a fraction, satisfies the relationship $N(1 - PR)\,(ID) = N(PR)\,(TD)$ or

$$(1 - PR)\,(ID) = (PR)\,(TD), \qquad (18)$$

where TD stands for the termination density in the prevalence pool, i.e., for the number of case terminations (by cure or death) divided by the case-time of experience in which they occurred. In the equilibrium state $TD = 1/\bar{D}$, the inverse of the mean duration of the illness. Substitution of this into equation 18 yields, as the static-state relationship of prevalence to incidence density,

$$PR = (ID)\bar{D}/[1 + (ID)\bar{D}]. \qquad (19)$$

As a deduction, then, the prevalence-odds are simply

$$(PR)/(1 - PR) = (ID)\bar{D}; \qquad (20)$$

and furthermore, for a comparison of the exposed (subscript 1) to the non-exposed (subscript 0), the prevalence-odds ratio (POR) is

$$POR = [(PR_1)/(1 - PR_1)]/[(PR_0)/(1 - PR_0)]$$

$$= (ID_1)\bar{D}_1/(ID_0)\bar{D}_0 \qquad (21)$$

$$= IDR \text{ if } \bar{D}_1 = \bar{D}_0 .$$

Thus, in a static population, the prevalence-odds ratio is estimable in the same terms as the incidence density ratio—through the exposure-odds ratio between the cases and the referents, without any rarity-assumption (cf. section 3). And again, if both of the exposure-specific prevalences are low, the prevalence-odds ratio is approximately equal to the prevalence ratio itself.

Now consider a limited category of age. Even if the population of interest in such a category can be thought of as static (with turnover) over time, and usually this is the case, the prevalence for it is not represented by formula 19 with the ordinary meaning for incidence density and duration. Instead, if that formula were to be used, the tally of incident cases in any given period of time would have to include the ones that enter the age-specific prevalence pool as carryover cases from the previous category of age; also, the mean duration of the illness should be adjusted downward to reflect those terminations within the category which result from cases reaching the upper bound of the category. The implementation of these considerations, in terms of formula 19 or otherwise, does not lead to any simple expression of wide applicability.

6. Example

Cole et al. identified all newly-diagnosed cases of bladder cancer in a (static) population (eastern Massachusetts) of known size over an 18-month period, drew a reference series from the source-population of the cases, and inquired (*inter alia*) into the subjects' histories with respect to cigarette-smoking (4). Some of the data (7) are presented in table 1.

The data allow the computation of age-specific overall incidence densities. For example, for the 50- to 54-years category the value is $35/(77,400)$ (1.5 years) $= 30/10^5$ years (cf. formulas 1 and 2). Actually this result ought to be corrected by allowing for prevalent cases (formula 5), but such a correction, which would be negligible in magnitude, is not feasible, because preva-

lent cases were excluded without tally in the selection of the reference series. The age-specific values obtained within the study are in close conformity with those derived (without prevalence correction) from the cancer registry of a neighboring region (Connecticut) a few years earlier (8). The latter data, too, are shown in table 1.

The samples of cases and noncases in each category of age allow the estimation of the corresponding incidence density ratio (without any rarity-assumption). For example, for the 50- to 54-years age category, the incidence density ratio (*IDR*)—i.e., the incidence density for smokers (ID_1) divided by that for nonsmokers (ID_0)—is estimated to be $\widehat{IDR} = (24/1)/(22/4) = 4.36$ (formula 3).

In order to provide for the estimation of absolute incidence density separately for smokers and nonsmokers, and as a matter of interest in its own right, the age-specific estimates for the etiologic fraction (with $IDR \geq 1$) or the preventive fraction ($\widehat{IDR} < 1$) are computed next. Thus, for the 50- to 54-years category age, for which $\widehat{IDR}$ ($= 4.36$) > 1, the etiologic fraction is estimated as follows: $\widehat{EF} = [(4.36 - 1)/4.36]24/25 = 0.74$ (formula 8). For the 60- to 64-years category $\widehat{IDR}$ ($= 0.49$) < 1, and therefore the preventive fraction is calculated (without inferring prevention): $\widehat{PF} = (1 - 0.49)$ $(31/36)/[(1 - 31/36)$ $(0.49) + 31/36] = 0.47$ (formula 11).

The incidence density estimates specific for the exposed and the non-exposed are then computed by the use of either formulas 6 and 7 (if $\widehat{IDR} \geq 1$) or formulas 9 and 10 (if $\widehat{IDR} < 1$). For the 50- to 54-years category the estimate for smokers is (4.36) $(30/10^5$ years) $(1 - 0.74) = 34/10^5$ years (formula 6), while the corresponding result for nonsmokers is $(30/10^5$ years) $(1 - 0.74) = 8/10^5$ years (formula 7). In the 60- to 64-years category the estimate for smokers is 0.49 $(56/10^5$ years)$/(1 - 0.47) = 52/10^5$ years (formula 9), while for nonsmokers it is $(56/10^5$ years)$/(1 - 0.47) = 110/10^5$ years.

Turning to the assessment of risk, con-

232   OLLI MIETTINEN

TABLE 1

Case-referent data by Cole et al. (4) and Cole (7) relating the incidence of bladder cancer to cigarette-smoking in men of various ages. The study involved complete ascertainment of newly-diagnosed cases in a population (eastern Massachusetts) of known size by age. Interviews were confined to a sample of cases as well as of non-cases. See section 6.

Age (years)	No. of new cases within 18 months	Size of source population in 10^a	Overall incidence density* in $(10^5 \text{ years})^{-1}$		No. of study subjects				Incidence density ratio	Smoking-related fraction of cases		Exposure-specific incidence density in $(10^5 \text{ years})^{-1}$	
			Study	Connecticut region (8)	Cases		Referents			Etiologic	Preventive	Sm. +	Sm. −
					Sm. + †	Sm. −	Sm. +	Sm. −					
50-54	35	77.4	30	(29)	24	1	22	4	4.36	.74		34	8
55-59	52	68.4	51	(48)	35	2	35	4	2.00	.47		54	27
60-64	52	61.5	56	(65)	31	5	38	3	.49		.48	52	110
65-69	86	47.4	120	(130)	46	7	42	15	2.35	.50		140	60
70-74	105	38.0	180	(170)	60	13	51	28	2.53	.50		230	90
75-79	76	23.2	220	(200)	39	14	32	20	1.74	.31		260	150

30-year risk at age 50 years given survival from other illness:

Smokers: $\hat{R}_{50,80} \doteq [(34 + 54 + 52 + 140 + 230 + 260)/10^5 \text{ years}] (5 \text{ years}) = 0.0385 = 3.9$ per cent.

Nonsmokers: $\hat{R}_{50,80} \doteq [(8 + 27 + 110 + 60 + 90 + 150)/10^5 \text{ years}] (5 \text{ years}) = 0.0223 = 2.2$ per cent.

Risk ratio estimate: $\hat{R}R_{50,80} = 3.85/2.23 = 1.7$

Risk difference estimate: $\hat{R}D_{50,80} = (3.85 - 2.23)$ per cent $= 1.6$ per cent.

* Two-digit accuracy.

† Sm+ and Sm−: smoker and nonsmoker, respectively.

sider the 30-year risk of bladder cancer for a 50-year-old man, assuming that without bladder cancer he would survive that period. If the man is a smoker, then the estimate is $\hat{R}_{50,80} = 1 - \exp \{ - [(34 + 54 + 52 + 140 + 230 + 260)/10^5 \text{ years}]5 \text{ years}\} = 1 - \exp(-0.0385) = 1 - \text{antil}_e(-0.0385) = 3.8$ per cent (formulas 16 and 13). Almost the same result can be obtained more simply from the approximate expression in formula 15. For a nonsmoker the corresponding estimate is 2.2 per cent. The estimate of the 30-year risk ratio at age 50 years is, then, 3.8/2.2 = 1.7, and the corresponding risk difference estimate is (3.8 − 2.2) per cent = 1.6 per cent.

7. Statistical aspects

7.1. Point estimation. As was illustrated in the above example, the various parametric relationships that were set forth provide for straight-forward point estimation of the various parameters of most direct interest. In the expressions for those parameters, the component parameters were simply replaced by their "sample values." This is essentially tantamount to maximum-likelihood estimation, with all its desirable properties, in large samples in particular.

7.2. Interval estimation. For incidence density ratio at any given age, large-sample $100(1-\alpha)$ per cent two-sided confidence limits ($\underline{IDR}$ and $\overline{IDR}$) may be set simply as

$$\underline{IDR}, \overline{IDR} = (\widehat{IDR})^{1 \pm g_{\alpha/2}/\chi}, \quad (22)$$

where $g_{\alpha/2}$ is the $100(1 - \alpha/2)$ percentile of the standard Gaussian distribution, and where χ is the positive square root of the 1 d.f. chi square statistic for significance testing of the association (9). The chi may derive from the ordinary test for a single two-by-two table or from the Mantel-Haenszel procedure (10). Correspondingly, the point estimate ($\widehat{IDR}$) is either the "cross-product ratio" from a single two-by-two table (1) or an appropriate estimate based on multiple tables (11). The limits

for the incidence density ratio are also the limits for the instantaneous risk ratio.

For the risk ratio from age a' to age a'' the limits may be set in an analogous manner:

$$\underline{RR}_{a',a''}, \overline{RR}_{a',a''} = (\widehat{RR}_{a',a''})^{1 \pm g_{\alpha/2}/\chi}. \quad (23)$$

The chi still derives from the overall significance test. For example, if limits were to be set for the risk ratio for which the point estimate was derived in table 1 and section 6, the chi value would be computed in terms of the Mantel-Haenszel test statistic (10) for the totality of age-specific two-by-two tables for which the data are given in table 1.

For the corresponding risk difference (RD) the limits may be taken as

$$\underline{RD}_{a',a''}, \overline{RD}_{a',a''} = (\widehat{RD})(1 \pm g_{\alpha/2}/\chi). \quad (24)$$

For the etiologic and preventive fractions the upper confidence bound cannot exceed unity, while the lower bound must be zero when $g_{\alpha/2} = \chi$ (and also when $g_{\alpha/2} > \chi$). Those constraints suggest the use of the limits

$$\underline{EF}, \overline{EF} = 1 - (1 - \widehat{EF})^{1 \pm g_{\alpha/2}/\chi}$$
$$(\text{with } \underline{EF} \geq 0) \quad (25)$$

and

$$\underline{PF}, \overline{PF} = 1 - (1 - \widehat{PF})^{1 \pm g_{\alpha/2}/\chi}$$
$$(\text{with } \underline{PF} \geq 0). \quad (26)$$

As to the incidence density among the exposed (formulas 6 and 9) or the non-exposed (formulas 7 and 10) the limits may be set as

$$\underline{ID}_i, \overline{ID}_i = (\widehat{ID}_i) \exp(\pm g_{\alpha/2}\hat{V}_i^{1/2}), \quad (27)$$

$i = 1, 0$, where $\hat{V}_i$ is the variance estimate of the natural logarithm of $\widehat{ID}_i$. This variance estimate may be taken as

$$\hat{V}_i = \hat{V} + [\ln(\widehat{ID}_i) - \ln(\widehat{ID})]^2/\chi^2, \quad (28)$$

where $\hat{V}$ is the variance estimate for the natural logarithm of the estimated overall incidence density ($\widehat{ID}$), computable as

$$\hat{V} = 1/(a'' + b''), \quad (29)$$

i.e., as the inverse of the total number of cases involved in the estimate.

Finally consider confidence limits for the exposure-specific risks, such as the ones examined in table 1 and section 6. In the usual situation, in which the risks are quite low, the limits may be taken as

$$\underline{R}_i, \overline{R}_i = \hat{R}_i \exp\left(\pm g_{\alpha/2} \hat{V}_i^{1/2}\right), \quad (30)$$

where $\hat{V}_i$ is an estimate of the variance of the natural logarithm of the point estimate. For the overall risk (formulas 13 and 15) one may use

$$\hat{V} = \Sigma_j [(\widehat{ID}_j)^2/(a''_j + b''_j)](w_j)^2/\hat{R}^2, \quad (31)$$

where $a''_j + b''_j$ is the number of cases on which ID_j is based. For the exposed and the non-exposed, the corresponding variances may be taken as

$$\hat{V}_i = \hat{V} + (\ln \hat{R}_i - \ln \hat{R})^2/\chi^2, \quad (32)$$

$i = 1, 0$. Here the χ^2 is still the 1 d.f. chi square statistic (10) for testing the hypothesis of no association.

Example. As an illustration of interval estimation of risk, consider again the data in table 1 and section 6, specifically the 30-year risk at age 50 years. The point estimate of the overall risk according to formula 13 (and 16) is $\hat{R} = 1 - \exp\{- [(30 + 51 + 56 + 120 + 180 + 220)/10^5 \text{ years}] 5 \text{ years}\} = 1 - \exp(-0.0329) = 3.2$ per cent. For the variance of its logarithm the estimate (formula 31) is $\hat{V} = \{[(30^2)/35 + \ldots + (220)^2/76]/(10^5 \text{ years})^2\}$ $(5 \text{ years})^2/(0.0323)^2 = 0.0030$. The corresponding 95 per cent confidence limits (formula 30) are, then, $\underline{R}, \overline{R} = (0.032) \exp [\pm 1.96(0.0030)^{1/2}] = 2.9$ per cent, 3.6 per cent. For the Mantel-Haenszel chi square, consider the exposed cases; the observed number is $24 + \ldots + 39 = 235$, while the expectation (10) and variance (10) are 220.4 and 22.12, respectively, giving $\chi^2 = (235 - 220.4)^2/22.1 = 9.6$. Thus, with risk estimates $R_1 = 3.8$ per cent and $R_0 = 2.2$ per cent (section 6), the variance estimate for the logarithm of the risk for smokers (formula 32) is $\hat{V}_1 = 0.0030 + (\ln 0.038 - \ln 0.032)^2/9.6 = .0061$, so that $\hat{V}_1^{1/2} = 0.078$. With this, the 95 per cent confidence limits (formula 30)

are (3.8 per cent) exp $[\pm 1.96(0.078)] = 3.3$ per cent, 4.4 per cent.

REFERENCES

1. Cornfield, J: A method of estimating comparative rates from clinical data. Application to cancer of the lung, breast and cervix. J Natl Cancer Inst 11:1269–1275, 1951
2. MacMahon B, Pugh TF: Epidemiology: Principles and Methods. Boston, Little, Brown and Co, 1970, chapter 12
3. Salber EJ, Trichopoulos D, MacMahon B: Lactation and reproductive histories of breast cancer patients in Boston, 1965–66. J Natl Cancer Inst 43:1013–1024, 1969
4. Cole P, Monson RR, Haning H, et al: Smoking and cancer of the lower urinary tract. N Engl J Med 284:129–134, 1971
5. Miettinen OS: Proportion of disease caused or prevented by a given exposure, trait or intervention. Am J Epidemiol 99:325–332, 1974
6. Chiang CL: Introduction to Stochastic Processes in Biostatistics. New York, John Wiley & Sons, Inc, 1968, chapter 12
7. Cole P: Personal communication, 1975
8. International Union Against Cancer: Cancer Incidence in Five Continents, Vol. 2. New York, Springer-Verlag, 1970
9. Miettinen, OS: Simple interval estimation of risk ratio. Am J Epidemiol 100:(Abs) 515–516, 1974
10. Mantel N, Haenszel W: Statistical aspects of the analysis of data from retrospective studies of disease. J Natl Cancer Inst 22:710–748, 1959
11. Gart, J: The comparison of proportions: a review of significance tests, confidence intervals and adjustments for stratification. Rev Int Statist Inst 39:148–169, 1971

APPENDIX 1

Test-based confidence limits

Ordinarily, large-sample confidence limits for a parameter (π) are set as

$$\underline{\pi}, \bar{\pi} = f^{-1}[f(\hat{\pi}) \pm g_{\alpha/2}(SE_{f(\hat{\pi})})]. \quad (A.1)$$

The transformation function (f) is chosen with the aim of attaining a Gaussian and stable-variance sampling distribution for the metameter $(f(\hat{\pi}))$ of the point estimate $(\hat{\pi})$; and the standard error, SE, is usually computed as a first-order Taylor series approximation, i.e., as $(SE_{\hat{\pi}})f'(\hat{\pi})$.

In the context of the estimates dealt with in the above, the formulation of the standard error according to the ordinary principles would tend to involve substantial complexity. At the same time, point estimation and significance-testing are quite simple.

This suggests the computation of the standard error from the point estimate and the test statistic. The rationale of this approach may not be completely transparent in the results offered, and some explanatory remarks may therefore be in order.

Consider first a parameter (π) with an expressly known null value (π_0) corresponding to the absence of any association between the exposure and the illness, i.e., a parameter such as rate ratio ($\pi_0 = 1$), rate difference ($\pi_0 = 0$) or etiologic fraction ($\pi_0 = 0$). Given that the metameter is successfully chosen (*vide supra*),

$$[f(\hat{\pi}) - f(\pi_0)]^2/[SE_{f(\hat{\pi})}]^2 = \chi^2 \quad (A.2)$$

if $\pi = \pi_0$, the chi square having one degree of freedom. Solving this for the standard error and substituting the result to formula A.1 yields

$$\underline{\pi}, \bar{\pi} = f^{-1}\{f(\hat{\pi}) \pm g_{\alpha/2}[f(\hat{\pi}) - f(\pi_0)]/\chi\}, \quad (A.3)$$

where χ is a square root (positive or negative) of χ^2. Finally, the chi value in this formulation may in fact be obtained from the Mantel-Haenszel statistic (10), which bears on the same null hypothesis. This principle underlies formulas 22–26, with no transformation in formula 24, and with the transformation $f(\cdot) = \ln[1 - (\cdot)]$ in formulas 25 and 26, the inverse function being $f^{-1}(\cdot) = 1 - \exp(\cdot)$.

When the null value is not firmly known, as when dealing with absolute exposure-specific rates or risks (formulas 27 and 30), formula A.1 is still used. Here the computation of the standard error is somewhat more complicated. We have, analogously with formula A.2,

$$[f(\hat{\pi}_1) - f(\hat{\pi}_0)]^2 / [SE_{f(\hat{\pi}_1)-f(\hat{\pi}_0)}]^2 = \chi^2, \quad (A.4)$$

with the subscripts referring to the exposed and non-exposed respectively, as before. But equivalently,

$$[f(\hat{\pi}_i) - f(\hat{\pi})]^2 / [SE_{f(\hat{\pi}_i)-f(\hat{\pi})}]^2 = \chi^2, \quad (A.5)$$

$i = 1, 0$, where $\hat{\pi}$ is the overall estimate for the exposed ($i=1$) and non-exposed ($i=0$) combined. As a further modification,

$$[f(\hat{\pi}_i) - f(\hat{\pi})]^2/\{[SE_{f(\hat{\pi}_i)}]^2 - [SE_{f(\hat{\pi})}]^2\} = \chi^2, \quad (A.6)$$

since $[SE_{f(\hat{\pi}_i)}]^2 = [SE_{f(\hat{\pi}_i) - f(\hat{\pi})}]^2 + [SE_{f(\hat{\pi})}]^2$. This implies that

$$SE_{f(\hat{\pi}_i)} = \{[SE_{f(\hat{\pi})}]^2 + [f(\hat{\pi}_i) - f(\hat{\pi})]^2/\chi^2\}^{1/2}. \quad (A.7)$$

as in formulas 28 and 32.

As to the choice of the metameter, the square root transformation might be preferred to the logarithmic one in formulas 27 and 30. This would imply

$$\underline{\pi}_i, \bar{\pi}_i = \{\hat{\pi}_i^{1/2} \pm g_{\alpha/2}[(SE_{\hat{\pi}})^2/4\hat{\pi} + (\hat{\pi}_i^{1/2} - \pi^{1/2})^2/\chi^2]^{1/2}\}^2. \quad (A.8)$$

ERI

ISBN 0-917227-02-6